Leishmaniasis in Sri Lanka

Leishmaniasis in Sri Lanka: A Research Review presents a unique and interesting scientific problem: *Leishmania donovani*–induced cutaneous leishmaniasis (CL). This new clinical entity is increasingly reported in many countries at present. This book presents the story of leishmaniasis in Sri Lanka through the author's 20-year experience. Through its comprehensive 13 chapters and over 270 references, the book sheds crucial light on the past, present, and future of leishmaniasis in the island, while covering historical aspects, progression in research on parasite, vector, host, immunology, clinical, diagnostic, treatment, patient care, and their corresponding trends. The content builds gradually to a final discussion of the gaps in knowledge, research needs, capacity building, and a model to manage an emerging health issue in a country. This concise yet comprehensive book is an ideal thought-provoking reference guide to professionals with a keen interest in the field of leishmaniasis.

Key Features

- Provides a comprehensive and complete resource on leishmaniasis, including various aspects of the disease, distilling credible information from available literature coupled with historical references.
- Follows a model approach for handling emerging infectious diseases for the benefit of clinicians and front-line workers.
- Discusses the unique problem of skin-localizing visceralizing parasites of *Leishmania* and provides basic principles of management for other infectious diseases and vector-borne infections.

Leishmaniasis in Sri Lanka
A Research Review

Yamuna Deepani Siriwardana

Professor
Head, Department of Parasitology,
Head, Parasitic Disease Research Unit,
Faculty of Medicine,
University of Colombo, Sri Lanka

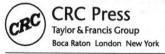

CRC Press
Taylor & Francis Group
Boca Raton London New York

CRC Press is an imprint of the
Taylor & Francis Group, an **informa** business

First edition published 2023
by CRC Press
6000 Broken Sound Parkway NW, Suite 300, Boca Raton, FL 33487-2742

and by CRC Press
4 Park Square, Milton Park, Abingdon, Oxon, OX14 4RN

CRC Press is an imprint of Taylor & Francis Group, LLC

Library of Congress Cataloging-in-Publication Data
Names: Siriwardana, Yamuna Deepani, author.
Title: Leishmaniasis in Sri Lanka : a research review / by Dr Yamuna Deepani Siriwardana.
Description: First edition. | Boca Raton, FL : CRC Press, 2023. | Includes bibliographical references and index. | Summary: "This focus reports a unique problem as leishmaniasis is caused by a new genetically modified parasite which is being increasingly reported in many other settings transforming into a global concern. It covers important aspects of the disease, priorities, gaps and challenges to enthuse professionals practicing in resource-limited settings"—Provided by publisher.
Identifiers: LCCN 2022025773 (print) | LCCN 2022025774 (ebook) |
ISBN 9781032251455 (hardback) | ISBN 9781032251479 (paperback) | ISBN 9781003281801 (ebook)
Subjects: MESH: Leishmaniasis | Neglected Diseases | Leishmania–pathogenicity | Sri Lanka
Classification: LCC RC153 (print) | LCC RC153 (ebook) | NLM WR 350 |
DDC 616.9/364–dc23/eng/20220701
LC record available at https://lccn.loc.gov/2022025773
LC ebook record available at https://lccn.loc.gov/2022025774

ISBN: 9781032251455 (hbk)
ISBN: 9781032251479 (pbk)
ISBN: 9781003281801 (ebk)

DOI: 10.1201/9781003281801

Typeset in Times
by codeMantra

Dedicated to all hardworking researchers who make the world beautiful.

Contents

Foreword

The author of this book is a recognized authority who has pioneered the investigation of leishmaniasis in Sri Lanka since the early 2000s. Reflected vividly in her writing is a high spirit of great enthusiasm and optimism, fostering her unrelenting effort of devotion to this greatly neglected disease that is emerging or re-emerging in her home island. Dr. Yamuna Deepani Siriwardana is undoubtedly an observant, thoughtful, and highly productive investigator in her chosen endeavour of research and education in clinico-epidemiology and public health. On display is her eminent role as a leader in organizing colleagues for education of professionals and general public as well as seeking outside support for resources and expertise in cutting-edge approaches toward the resolution of problems at hand. She is keenly recognized as indispensable under resource-scarce conditions. Putting this recognition into practice has contributed significantly to her accomplishments, as documented in the well-organized and informative chapters of this book. Readers of the next generation are expected to find this book inspirational for charting a path to success of their own through self-sufficiency with boundless passion as Dr. Siriwardana has achieved in fighting the adversity of leishmaniasis.

Kwang Poo Chang
Professor of Microbiology/Immunology
Center for Cancer Biology. Immunology and Infection
Chicago Medical School
Rosalind Franklin University of Medicine and Science
North Chicago, Illinois, USA

Preface

New disease foci and changing scenarios are frequently reported in leishmaniasis. Empowering the different stakeholder groups in affected countries is of prime importance in combatting the disease. Raising public and professional awareness is another responsibility of those who discover information. A series of ten books was written with the aim of informing and motivating newcomers in different stakeholder groups, including academics, clinicians, researchers, laboratory managers, research laboratory workers, clinical laboratory technicians, primary healthcare workers, and general public.

Posing a threat to the regional drive for leishmaniasis elimination in the Indian subcontinent, Sri Lanka reports one of the largest known epidemics of *L. donovani*–induced human cutaneous leishmaniasis (CL). Meanwhile, many complexities are also associated. This book presents the story of leishmaniasis in Sri Lanka, identifies its position in the global scale, and discusses information gaps and current needs in operational aspects. It is aimed at informing and motivating young researchers coming into the field of leishmaniasis in disease-emerging settings.

In Sri Lanka, the disease was almost unheard of in the past. The first locally transmitted case of the current outbreak was detected by us in 2001 in a soldier with a chronic undiagnosed facial lesion. Diagnosis enabled successful treatment, leaving us with much satisfaction, happiness, and an array of scientific questions.

This report paved the way for an interesting scientific journey. The patient was traced back, absence of overseas travel was confirmed, and we offered a series of disease awareness programmes in the patient area, resulting in detection of many more cases from the same locality. We were able to start the first leishmaniasis clinic and laboratory in the University of Colombo, and disease awareness programmes were extended to cover multiple professional sectors, and scientific research was begun in spite of scarce resources. Increasing patient numbers have been reported since then.

I also recall evaluating many thousands of such patients and discussing many problems faced by them. Conducting many awareness programmes under security cover from Sri Lanka Army in a war-affected area in Northern Sri Lanka (Vavuniya) and conducting the first field survey in the same area during a time of high political unrest were challenging but rewarding and interesting tasks that I undertook with no external instructions but for my own interest. These activities provided us with opportunities not only to explore the real context but to experience the difficulties faced by the inhabitants in these areas. Back home in Colombo, spending time talking to patients, following them up, observing how healing occurs, and informally observing changing disease patterns over the years had always interested me. Most of these observations led to scientific studies which subsequently confirmed the accuracy of such assumptions. Changing micro clinical patterns within existing main profiles, presence of silent visceral infection, presence of a high humoral response in skin infections, atypical leishmaniasis as a different clinical entity, and different and independent disease foci in North and South in Sri Lanka are some of them. We also had failures and deficiencies in what we were doing.

Comprehensive understanding of the present situation and accurate predictions of harmless or potentially dangerous occurrences are essential. Prioritizing actions on a time scale to gather information and utilizing the generated knowledge in operation, prioritization, and implementation of such action require a correct understanding of present context.

Emerging researchers have a great responsibility in training themselves and their followers. The outcome can be better when leadership originates from within the affected countries. It is important to understand how multifaceted approaches can be useful in dealing with a scientific problem. This is discussed in detail in a separate chapter.

Research, diagnosis, patient care, and disease control efforts spiced up with enthusiasm for all involved categories are extremely important to all leishmaniasis-beaten poor settings in the world. As a clinician and a researcher, I feel certainly committed to contribute to disease control efforts. I sincerely hope that the reader will enjoy as well as benefit from this series of books, will support further dissemination of the knowledge, and will take a minute to brainstorm on what should be and what could be done by each one of us before disease control becomes more difficult in our countries.

Yamuna Deepani Siriwardana, MBBS, PhD
Head, Department of Parasitology
Head, Parasitic Disease Research Unit
Faculty of Medicine
University of Colombo
Sri Lanka
https://www.res.cmb.ac.lk/parasitology/hvyd.siriwardena/

Acknowledgements

The academic within myself is a product of a team effort. I am indebted to countless people in local and global academia, and society.

My first encounter with a case of leishmaniasis was on my first day as a probationary lecturer in the university system. My knowledge in research and academia was almost zero. I remain very grateful to Professors MM Ismail (late), N.Karunaweera and R. Wickremasinghe for teaching me the ABCs of research and academia. I recall with deep gratitude my respected teachers and senior colleagues who mentored me through various do's and don'ts in the new position.

Local expertise or access to global information was also scarce. I faced many challenges at the beginning. I was fortunate to receive my Commonwealth Doctoral Scholarship and meet my first leishmaniasis teachers, globally renowned Dr. Michael Chance, Dr. Harry Noyes, and Dr. Nich Beeching of Liverpool University, and Professor Paul Bates of Lancaster University in the UK. They guided, inspired, and taught me the fundamentals of leishmaniasis. I would not have been able to lay an accurate foundation in research without their support.

Meeting my PhD examiner Professor Jeffrey Jon Shaw of Universidade de São Paulo, Brazil and getting very encouraging comments was a strong inspirational milestone during my early career. I remain grateful to Dr. Anuradha Dube of Central Drug Research Institute, India and Professor Mitali Chatterjee of the Institute of Postgraduate Medical Education and Research, India for visiting the home laboratory to establish many techniques and The World Academy of Sciences (TWAS) for awarding me a science exchange opportunity that enabled these visits. Guidance I receive from Professor Shyam Sundar, programme director of Kala-azar Medical Research Center in India on patient care and research has been invaluable in my development as a clinician. All these remain as inspirational high points in my academic life.

Supportive funding authorities not only supported research but assured me of the accuracy of my pathway as a junior researcher. I am indebted forever to Sri Lanka Army for saving my life! Without their security support during many visits to unsettled areas during a period of political unrest, initial findings on leishmaniasis would have been impossible. Many local and international institutions have provided immense support. Patients in different parts of the country have not only been supportive, but their inspiring words still echo in my heart.

I am eternally grateful to globally renowned senior researcher Professor KP Chang of Rosalind Franklin University of Medicine and Science, USA for his continued guidance and support. I found a great teacher, dedicated mentor, and an effective collaborator for life in him. I am grateful to Professor KP Chang for his valuable comments on this work and for providing the Foreword to the book. I am extremely thankful to global experts in the field of leishmaniasis Professors Shyam Sundar, David Sacks, and Drs Byron Arana and Anuradha Dube for reviewing a book in this series. These books are under publication.

I am indebted to my clinical teacher Dr. Sarath Gaminie de Silva, senior consultant physician and former medical specialist of Ministry of Health Care and Nutrition, in Sri Lanka for his very valuable comments on this work. Technical assistance in photography was provided by the Audio Visual Unit of Faculty of Medicine, University of Colombo.

I am indebted to my parents, husband, and two daughters for their love and patience when I took many hundreds of days from their time for this work.

I thank the professional team including Ms Shivangi Pramanik, Ms Himani Dwivedi, and Ms Iris Fahrer of Taylor & Francis/CRC Press Group, and Ms Sathya Devi of codeMantra for handling the publication process with style and efficiency.

Author

Professor Yamuna Deepani Siriwardana is a clinician, university academic, and researcher who also earned the first Sri Lankan PhD on leishmaniasis. She is the author of a series of ten books on leishmaniasis written for different stakeholder groups in the field. She diagnosed the first case of the ongoing outbreak of the disease in Sri Lanka 20 years ago, with her team. Since then, she has pioneered many patient-care and research activities in her country, including establishment of the national awareness, first patient diagnostic service, research laboratory, and technician training programme for the country. Her work has resulted in many scientific publications and patent applications to her credit on leishmaniasis. She is also a recipient of many scientific awards including Commonwealth Doctoral Scholarship award in UK, a young affiliate fellowship of The World Academy of Sciences (TWAS), presidential awards, orations, and many other awards for scientific research. She currently serves as a teacher, a post-graduate trainer, and a researcher in leishmaniasis.

Author

Abbreviations

ACD	Active Case Detection
AtCL	Atypical Lesions in Cutaneous Leishmaniasis
AnCL	Anthroponotic Cutaneous Leishmaniasis
APCD	Activated Passive Case Detection
CCL	Classical Cutaneous Leishmaniasis
CD	Cluster of Differentiation
CI	Confidence Interval
CL	Cutaneous Leishmaniasis
CO I	Cytochrome Oxidase subunit I
Cyt b	Cytochrome oxidase b
DCL	Diffuse Cutaneous Leishmaniasis
DDT	Dichloro Diphenyl Trichloroethane
FCS	Fetal Calf Serum
FGT	Formol Gel Test
HLA	Human Leukocyte Antigen
HS	Hypertonic Saline
IC-RDT	Immune-Chromatographic Rapid Diagnostic Test
IL-2	Interleukin-2
INF	Interferon
ITS2	Internal Transcribed Spacer 2
LAMP	Loop Mediated Isothermal Amplification
M 199	Medium 199
MHC	Major Histocompatibility Complex
ML	Mucosal Leishmaniasis
MLEE	Multi Locus Enzyme Electrophoresis
NF	Northern Focus
NIH	National Institute of Health
NK cells	Natural Killer cells
NNN medium	Novy, McNeal and Nicolle medium
NUTs	Non-Ulcerative Type
PCDs	Passive Case Detections
PG	Post-Graduate
6-PGDH	6-Phospo-Gluconate Dehydrogenase gene
PKDL	Post Kala-azar Dermal Leishmaniasis

PPV	Positive Predictive Value
PUO	Pyrexia of Unknown Origin
RFHT	Radio Frequency-induced Heat Therapy
SEA	South East Asian
SF	Southern Focus
SNPs	Single Nucleotide Polymorphisms
spp.	Species
SSG	Sodium StiboGluconate
TNF	Tumour Necrosis Factor
UCFM	Faculty of Medicine of the University of Colombo
UG	Under Graduate
UTs	Ulcerative Types
VL	Visceral Leishmaniasis

OTHER BOOKS UNDER PUBLICATION ON LEISHMANIASIS BY THE AUTHOR

1. *An Overview on Leishmaniasis: Review of Essential Literature for the Emerging Professionals*
2. *Clinician's Essential Guide on Visceral Leishmaniasis in a Focus of Dermotropic L. donovani Infection (Based on Sri Lankan Experience)*
3. *Establishing Your Leishmaniasis Research Laboratory: A Guide Book for Emerging Laboratory Managers in Resource Limited Settings*
4. *Young Researcher's Essential Protocols in Leishmaniasis: For Emerging Clinical and Research Laboratories in Resource Limited Settings*
5. *Laboratory Diagnosis of Leishmaniasis: For Routine Hospital Laboratories in Leishmaniasis Endemic Settings*
6. *Becoming a Field Leader: A Visionary Approach for Primary Health Care Workers in Leishmaniasis Endemic Settings*
7. *Essential Facts in Field Screening and Combatting Leishmaniasis: For Public Health Inspectors and Midwives in Sri Lanka (Local Sinhala Language)*
8. *Let Us Know Leishmaniasis: Essential Facts for School Children*
9. *The Story of Leishmaniasis: Essential Facts for Sri Lankan School Children (Local Sinhala Language)*

History and Onset of the Epidemic

1

Leishmaniasis in Sri Lanka was sporadic and was limited to a few historical case reports in the past. Subsequently, a few imported cases were reported in the 1960s with a few locally acquired cases in the 1990s. Since then, the disease remained almost unheard of until 2001 when the index case was detected by us. Immediately following this, we conducted professional and public awareness programmes and established diagnostic facilities in the author's institution. These efforts resulted in the immediate reporting of many more cases of leishmaniasis from different localities in the island, indicating the long-term existence of a silent transmission cycle of leishmaniasis in the country. The first historical record on leishmaniasis in colonial Sri Lanka was made in 1904. This was followed by the report of many thousands of patients whose diagnosis was attributed to leishmaniasis in the next few decades. Further confirming this finding parasitological studies have favoured a long-term existence and a genetic variation of *Leishmania* in the island.

This book presents the story of leishmaniasis in Sri Lanka including the onset, progression, current status, gaps, and future needs.

1.1 HISTORICAL CASES

Leishmaniasis could preferably be identified as a recently reported health threat in the island. However, it is interesting to note some historical cases of parasitologically proven leishmaniasis in the island. The first formal record was available in 1904 on a case of leishmaniasis (Perry, 1904). Information contained in this report could be considered adequate to support the said conclusions. Following this, several government reports presented by the British in colonial Sri Lanka since 1928 had indicated the occurrence of cutaneous

DOI: 10.1201/9781003281801-1

leishmaniasis in many thousands of patients (Bridger, 1928; Briercliffe, 1930). Deaths have also been reported under this category leading to strong suspicion on the possibility of an alternate diagnosis since death due to leishmanial infections on the skin are extremely rare. Furthermore, details on clinical presentations or how they confirmed the clinical diagnoses are also not available. It is rather possible that similar tropical conditions were diagnosed to be cases of cutaneous leishmaniasis and increased the total case numbers to a very high level while the actual case burden remained somewhat low in this setting. Meanwhile, it may be justifiable to assume that leishmaniasis had probably been considered as the diagnosis in these patients since the condition would have been reported in other British colonies including India and African settings during that time. However, more reliable formal records on the occurrence of leishmaniasis in Sri Lanka are available in the more recent past (Athukorale et al., 1992; Dissanaike, 1981; Naotunne et al., 1990; Seneviratne et al., 1995). The forthcoming sections summarize these historical reports.

1.1.1 Case 1 (H1): A Northern Sri Lankan or an Indian Immigrant? Anergic CL or Post Kala-Azar Dermal Leishmaniasis?

In the 1960s, CL was confirmed by microscopy in a patient from Northern Sri Lanka who presented with skin nodules. He had no overseas travel history. The lesions were attributed to anergic CL caused by a dermotropic species of *Leishmania* other than *L. donovani*, probably due to decreased immunity levels. However, it is interesting to note that the author, Prof. Dissanaike, suspected post-kala-azar dermal leishmaniasis in this patient. He was suspected to be an illegal immigrant from India, merely since VL was not heard locally. This case was reported later in 1981 (Dissanaike, 1981) (Figure 1.1).

1.1.2 Case 2 (H2): Suspicion of Visceral Disease (1960)

Again, in the 1960s, classical signs of visceral leishmaniasis (VL) were reported in a British girl who had a travel history of 6 weeks in Sri Lanka, 1 year prior to the onset of her clinical features. Bone marrow examination revealed *Leishmania* species amastigotes. She had multiple, but short (less than an hour) stops in Rome, Bombay, Cairo, Bahrain, and Tehran during her journey from the UK to Sri Lanka and back. Probably due to the fact that some

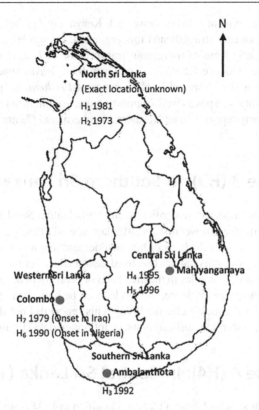

FIGURE 1.1 Spatial distribution of the historical cases of leishmaniasis in Sri Lanka (1973–1996).

of these places had reported leishmaniasis and it was not heard of in Sri Lanka at that time, it was concluded that she probably acquired leishmaniasis during one of these stops. This case was reported in 1973 (Chapman, 1973).

Both 1973 and 1981 reports indicate the occurrence of visceralizing and probably PKDL-causing strains of *Leishmania* in Sri Lanka for a long time. However, local transmission was not suspected due to lack of reported cases during that time. Meanwhile, it is interesting to note the valuable predictions made by Prof. A.S. Dissanaike on the possibility of a silent sylvatic cycle in Sri Lanka (Dissanaike, 1981), though these views have not been taken forward by subsequent groups. However, later on, with formal reporting of some local cases, scientists suspected a silent sylvatic cycle and indigenous transmission in Sri Lanka (Wijesundera, 2001). Interestingly, the possibility of a genetic variant of *L. donovani* causing CL in the country was not even thought of. That may be the probable reason to conclude the imported nature of H1 and H2.

Then, available evidence from India and Kenya on *Leishmania tropica*–induced VL obviously strengthened this argument, though H1 and H2 would have been the early signs of indigenous transmission of *L. donovani*–induced CL. Incomplete evidence for visceralization in these leaves space to hypothesize long-term and widespread local existence of *Leishmania* species, resulting in different phenotypes as well. Supporting this argument, a few more cases were subsequently reported from Northern, Southern, and Central provinces in Sri Lanka (Figure 1.1).

1.1.3 Case 3 (H3): In Southern Sri Lanka (1992)

In 1992, CL was reported in a patient from Ambalantota Southern Sri Lanka who lacked an overseas travel history (Athukorale et al., 1992). The patient had an ulcerated lesion over the back of his shoulder and diagnosis was confirmed by light microscopy. This patient had lived near a river, but any evidence of a close association with jungles in the area had not been elicited. The patient had provided contradictory evidence, though later on he had admitted an association with jungles (Killick Kendrik, 1996). This report did not describe treatment response, systemic manifestations, or follow-up data (Figure 1.1).

1.1.4 Case 4 (H4): In Central Sri Lanka (1994)

Another locally acquired case of CL was identified in 1994 from Mahiyangana in the Uva province in Central Sri Lanka (Seneviratne et al., 1995). The patient had two lesions over his back and face. Diagnosis was confirmed by microscopy in one lesion that subsequently responded to liquid nitrogen therapy. This patient lived in close proximity to jungles, had a daily outdoor routine, and slept outside on hot days. He spent weekends in Badulla, a location in the same province (Figure 1.1).

1.1.5 Case 5 (H5): An Unreported Case from Central Sri Lanka (1996)

Two years later, another locally acquired case of microscopically confirmed CL was identified in the Central province from a place about 11 miles away from the place where the 1994 case spent the weekends (Killick-Kendrick, 1996). The patient had a history of working in the Middle East 5 years prior to the onset of lesions. He also had jungle-associated routines for gem mining in his residential area in Sri Lanka (Figure 1.1).

1.1.6 Cases 6 and 7 (H6 and H7): Imported Cases from Colombo

In 1990, two more imported cases were reported (Naotunne et al., 1990). The first case was a school teacher who worked in Nigeria for 2 years. She noticed the lesions during her stay in Nigeria in 1980. She had facial and forearm lesions.

A second case was reported from Colombo during the same time. He was employed as a truck driver in Iraq in 1979. During the fifth month of employment, he had noticed the lesions on his back. The lesions responded well to treatment. However, they reappeared 2 years later, upon his return to Sri Lanka. He presented for medical care in 1987 with a few satellite lesions that appeared later around the non-healing ulcer.

Diagnosis was confirmed by both microscopy and *in vitro* cultivation of the lesion material in both cases. Both were suspected to be imported cases which were supported by clinical evidence that was compatible with self-healing *Leishmania major* infections occurring in Nigeria and dry, chronic lesions of *L. tropica* occurring in urban Iraq.

However, the remote possibility of local acquisition of infection and subsequent occurrence of clinical disease cannot be excluded. Proper local travel details or time maps are not available probably since authors did not consider this possibility (Figure 1.1).

1.2 RECENT EPIDEMIC IN THE NORTH

Almost a decade later in 2001, a soldier from Weli-Oya in Northern Sri Lanka was referred to us with a facial ulcer of 7-month duration. He had been investigated and treated for many other possibilities. The request was to exclude the possibility of any parasitic cause. Lesion scrapings demonstrated *Leishmania* spp. amastigotes in microscopy. Clinical evaluation confirmed CL without evidence for visceralization. There was no overseas travel.

This finding raised our suspicion on an already-established local transmission cycle of leishmaniasis in Sri Lanka, and activities to create disease awareness among professionals and general public immediately followed. The first programme was held in the Victory hospital in Anuradhapura (2001) in the patient area. Subsequent programmes covered military forces, police officers, home guard officers, school children, general public, medical professional, and para-medical staff of government hospitals under military cover in the Vavuniya region in war-affected Northern Sri Lanka (2002–2003). These efforts resulted in the detection of many more cases of locally acquired CL

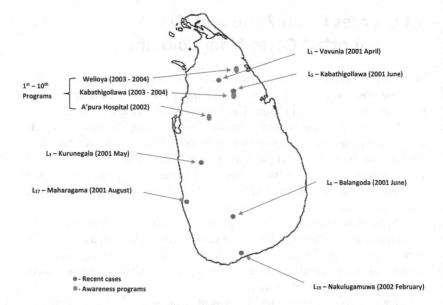

FIGURE 1.2   Locations of the awareness programmes (2001–2006) and reported cases of CL (L 1, 3, 5, 6, 17, and 49, 2001 April–2002 April) during the initial stages of the outbreak of leishmaniasis in Sri Lanka.

occurring in the same area. The majority were young adult male soldiers having close association with scrub jungles in the area (Siriwardana et al., 2003) (Figure 1.2).

1.3 EXPANSION OF CASE REPORTING

Increased case reporting necessitated development of our capacity in patient management. The country was not adequately equipped to handle such a situation. A weekly leishmaniasis patient care and microscopic diagnostic facility were immediately established in the Department of Parasitology, Faculty of Medicine in the University of Colombo. Meanwhile, the referring dermatologist who served a main hospital in Northern Sri Lanka (Anuradhapura) took up a new post in a main hospital in Southern Sri Lanka (Matara), which followed the detection of further cases from the South. Awareness efforts were further extended to cover Mamadala, Kataragama, and Dikwella, locations situated in Southern Sri Lanka. This ensured a continued flow of over

100 suspected patients. The diagnosis was confirmed in over 80% of them, with confirmation of indigenous transmission in all cases within the next 12 months.

Since then, cases of leishmaniasis have been continuously reported to hospitals and our own institution and later on to many other research settings in the country.

1.4 RESEARCH INTO THE RECENT EPIDEMIC

Formal studies were also begun. *In vitro* cultivation and molecular biological diagnostic techniques (PCR) were established in the Faculty of Medicine in the University of Colombo under the guidance of the leishmaniasis reference laboratory in University de Montpellier, France and Liverpool School of Tropical Medicine and Hygiene in the UK where the author was able to pursue molecular biological studies of a commonwealth doctoral training programme (Figure 1.3).

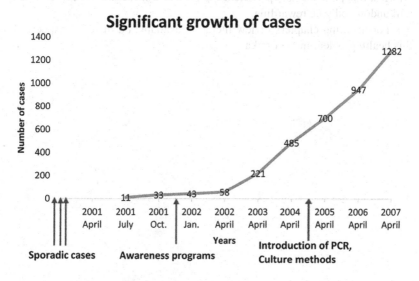

FIGURE 1.3 Exponential growth of the reported numbers of patients with CL during the initial stages (2001–2007) in Sri Lanka (authors data base on leishmaniasis).

Case reporting has continued since then. The work of the weekly leishmaniasis clinic in Colombo expanded under the Centre for Leishmaniasis Research, Training, and Diagnosis of the University of Colombo (https://med.cmb.ac.lk/parasitology/pdru/leishmaniasis/ctrdl/). Multiple research projects have been conducted, training programmes for medical and para-medical personnel have been established, and scientific information on the local situation of leishmaniasis has been produced, enabling the development of action guidelines for leishmaniasis control in Sri Lanka (Faculty of Medicine, Colombo, 2009).

Subsequently, other universities and research institutions in Sri Lanka initiated research on leishmaniasis. The research community has slowly grown in numbers, expertise, and physical capacity. A considerable volume of scientific information on the local problem has been produced through efforts made by these Sri Lankan scientists.

In spite of this, the epidemic has expanded in many dimensions, leaving much work for scientists. The primary responsibility in revealing hidden facts through proper scientific tools, prediction and identification of potential dangers, strengths and required action, and educating the different stakeholder categories lie on the local content experts. In fact, leishmaniasis in South Asia presents a complex picture that resembles a microcosm of the disease complex in the world (Chang et al., 2018). These are challenging and require great effort, skills, patience, and persistence to achieve a successful outcome, which will undoubtedly be rewarding.

Forthcoming chapters review literature available on different aspects of this health problem in Sri Lanka.

Attempts on Parasite Studies 2

The Unusual Parasite

2.1 NECESSITY FOR PARASITE IDENTIFICATION

Leishmaniasis is known to result from over 20 incriminated parasite species of *Leishmania* or *Viannia*, the two subgenera of the genus *Leishmania*. The clinical outcome takes three main forms, affecting skin (cutaneous leishmaniasis), mucosa (mucosal leishmaniasis), or internal organs (visceral leishmaniasis), mainly depending on the causative species (Dedet et al., 2009; Banuls et al., 2007). Other less influential factors in determining the clinical outcome include host genetics (Bucheton et al., 2003), patient nutritional level (El-Safi et al., 2002), ethnicity and origin (Ibrahim et al., 1999), age (Marty et al., 2007), vector (Bates, 2007), and parasite characteristics such as infective inoculum and the infecting body site (Lang et al., 2003; Almeida, 2002). Patient management, treatment response, transmission characteristics, and therefore preventive and control strategies depend largely on the causative agent. Therefore, it is imperative to characterize the causative species in a timely manner when leishmaniasis emerges at a new focus.

DOI: 10.1201/9781003281801-2

9

2.2 COMMENCEMENT OF PARASITOLOGICAL RESEARCH

This need was addressed immediately following the detection of the first few cases (Siriwardana et al., 2003). The technique of iso-enzyme characterization or multilocus enzyme electrophoresis (MLEE) was considered the gold standard in the species characterization in leishmaniasis. First attempts we made using the MLEE technique identified *Leishmania donovani* of zymodeme MON 37 as the local causative species (Karunaweera et al., 2003).

L. donovani is considered the most virulent parasite species, resulting in visceral leishmaniasis at a global scale. Cutaneous leishmaniasis caused by *L. donovani* is rare and infrequent (Sharma et al., 2005; Mebrahtu et al., 1993; Loo et al., 2005; Harms et al., 2003; Ben-Ami et al., 2002; Pratlong et al., 1995; Adler et al., 1966). Occasional reports on mucotropism (Mahdi et al., 2005; Sethuraman et al., 2008) and concurrent cutaneous lesions with visceral disease (Ben-Ami et al., 2002) have also been reported. Usually, dermotropic forms also tend to visceralize specially in the immune compromised status (Darcis et al., 2017; Blum-Dominguez et al., 2017). In addition, atypical cutaneous manifestations caused by *L. donovani* have also been reported from many countries, including India, Ethiopia, and Israel (Adler et al., 1966; Ponce et al., 1991; Mebrahtu et al., 1993; Pratlong et al., 1995; Schnur et al., 1977; Sharma et al., 2005).

Furthermore, a Sri Lankan study also revealed the first report of zymodeme MON-37 of *L. donovani* causing human CL. This zymodeme has only been isolated from sandflies and cases of human visceral leishmaniasis in India and Ethiopia (Gebre-Michael et al., 1996) and in Israel (Schnur et al., 2001; Moreno et al., 1986, 1989).

Isoenzyme profiles of MON-37 and MON-2 strains of *L. donovani* are closely related to each other, apart from the different mobility patterns of a single enzyme 6PGDH. Therefore, it was unusual and interesting that the Sri Lankan strain results in cutaneous disease, while the Indian strain remains the predominant cause of visceral leishmaniasis in a clear majority of cases in India. This finding also indicated possible unreliability of the technique in species determination.

Controversial evidence has been produced regarding MLEE, and this biochemical technique has been continuously challenged in the recent past by true genetic-based methods. Isoenzyme characterization is a technique introduced in the 1970s (Chance et al., 1974). MLEE examines the enzyme profile of the organism under study and enzyme mobility patterns in an electrically charged field. Organisms within the genus *Leishmania* are subdivided into species and strains by examining the mobility patterns of a group of iso-enzymes. Parasites are assigned to the main operational taxonomic unit (OTU) known as zymodemes based on the mobility patterns of iso-enzymes. MLEE does not always reflect the true genetic basis of the organism under study (Massamba et al., 1998; Moreno et al., 1986; Cupolillo et al., 1995; Alam et al., 2009; Kuhls et al., 2008). Genetic variation is already known to exist within the *Leishmania* parasites that belong to the same zymodeme (Reale et al., 2010). Genetic studies on zymodeme MON-37 of *L. donovani* have not really reflected the genetic or geographical basis of the said classification (Alam et al., 2009).

Meanwhile, cases of cutaneous leishmaniasis continued to be reported to the University's leishmaniasis clinic in Colombo. Contradictory evidence provided by the first research left us with a new challenge to either re-confirm or refute those findings using better methods.

Further studies commenced immediately following this finding. Employment of true genetic-based methods provided answers. The finding of *L. donovani* was further confirmed by the study of a partial gene sequence of the 6-phospogluconate dehydrogenase gene (6-PGDH) and reported in year 2007 (Siriwardana et al., 2007). Sri Lankan parasites were clearly different from *Leishmania tropica* and *L. major*, which are said to be the most related to the *L. donovani* complex. This evidence provided a strong background to conclude that Sri Lankan cutaneous leishmaniasis is caused by the *L. donovani* complex. Sri Lankan isolates were found in the most peripheral branches of the evolutionary tree, indicating the more recent evolution of them in comparison to other members of the genus *Leishmania*.

2.3 *L. DONOVANI* MON-2 AND *L. DONOVANI* MON-37

Sri Lankan *L. donovani* MON-37 isolates were further compared with those of the Indian *L. donovani* MON-2, the commonest zymodeme reported in India. DNA sequences of *L. donovani* MON-37 Sri Lankan sequence and that of *L. donovani* MON-2 and MON-18 sequences of Indian origin were converted into protein sequences. A single-nucleotide difference was responsible for the occurrence of an uncharged asparagine residue (codon AAC) in the MON-2 sequence, while a negatively charged aspartic acid residue (codon GAC) was detected in MON-1, MON-18, and MON-37 sequences. This single–base pair change resulted in a protein with lower mobility in the

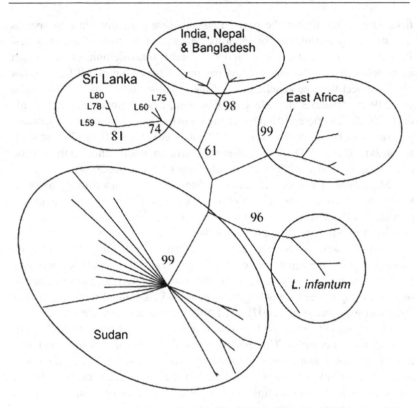

FIGURE 2.1 Analysis of the genetic relationship of *L. donovani* and *L. infantum* isolates from different geographical locations using partial sequencing of the 6-PGDH gene. (Data from Siriwardana HVYD et al., "*Leishmania donovani* and cutaneous leishmaniasis, Sri Lanka," *Emerging Infectious Diseases* 13 (3) (2007):476–8.)

MON-2 strain and differentiated it from the MON-37 strain, further highlighting the genetic similarities between Sri Lankan and Indian *L. donovani* (Siriwardana et al., 2007). In spite of this finding, the local clinical picture remained confined to cutaneous disease in increasing numbers of patients detected in Colombo. However, full-length sequences of these genes were not obtained in our study. Therefore, the possibility of changes occurring elsewhere was not excluded.

This situation again left the scientists with yet an unanswered third question. Are they genetically different from other known *L. donovani*? It was necessary to study the infra-specific strain variation to identify the differences and understand the origin of the local parasite. The *L. donovani* complex demonstrates a clear geographical relationship to their strain variation (Mauricio et al., 2001; Jamjoom et al., 2004; Zemanova et al., 2004; Quispe-Tintaya et al., 2005; Kuhls et al., 2005).

Therefore, a third component employing 16 *L. donovani*–specific genetic loci (micro satellite loci) that are known to demonstrate infra-specific variation within *L. donovani* was added to the study. This study placed local *L. donovani* in a distinct clade that is probably new and that differs from the Indian, Sudanese, and South African *L. donovani* species as well as from *Leishmania infantum*. This concluded that local cutaneous leishmaniasis is caused by a genetically distinct variant within the *L. donovani* complex (Siriwardana et al., 2007). Meantime, the study also demonstrated a close relationship of Sri Lankan isolates with those of the Indian subgroup (Figure 2.1).

To date, few more subsequent studies have confirmed our original finding of *L. donovani* based on the cytochrome b gene of *Leishmania* (Yatawara et al., 2008), microsatellite sequence typing (Alam et al., 2009, 2014), whole-genome sequencing (Zhang et al., 2014), and mini-circle kDNA (Kariyawasam et al., 2017).

Few years later, autochthonous visceral leishmanial infections were also identified in a few Sri Lankan patients (discussed in subsequent chapters). Studies on the causative species using MLEE has revealed *L. donovani* of zymodeme MON-37 as the responsible organism of visceral leishmaniasis in Sri Lanka (Ranasinghe et al., 2012). This observation raises the question of underlying mechanisms, leading to visceralization of some isolates, while a large proportion of infections caused by the same organism remain confined to the skin. This question is discussed in the forthcoming chapters.

Clinical Aspects 3

3.1 CUTANEOUS LEISHMANIASIS CONTINUE TO BE REPORTED

Some of our locally reported historical cases indicated the possible existence of leishmanial infections consistent with a clinical picture of cutaneous leishmaniasis (CL) since long. However, it is interesting to note the evidence provided by the rest of historical cases on the possibility of visceral leishmaniasis (VL) also occurring in this country. None of the reports, however, provided adequate evidence to confirm or refute the co-existence of both visceral and cutaneous manifestations or post-kala-azar dermal leishmaniasis (PKDL) in them. Subsequently, all the initial cases of the recent epidemic presented with skin lesions and appeared to be consistent with CL. Is this the only clinical form emerging or prevalent in this setting? What are the characteristics of CL in Sri Lanka? What are the sequelae of an infection caused by a genetically variant visceralizing parasite? Evidence-based information was necessary for case suspicion, diagnosis, and management in a community. Therefore, it was then necessary to study the clinical profile through scientific methods.

3.2 FIRST FORMAL STUDY IN YEAR 2003

The first clinical study on leishmaniasis in Sri Lanka was initiated in 2001, immediately following the detection of our index case in 2001 (Siriwardana et al., 2003). This was carried out as a descriptive study on the first 65 cases. The study group included those who were referred to us for diagnostic

DOI: 10.1201/9781003281801-3

confirmation. The majority were male soldiers of the young adult (21–40 years) age group. Skin lesions of these patients belonged to various stages of lesion development observed in classical cutaneous leishmaniasis (CCL), that is; acne-form papules of less than 1 cm diameter, larger nodules, ulcerating nodules, and completed ulcers. (Figure 3.1). Atypical manifestations (Figure 3.2) were not noticed in these patients. The lesions mainly occurred on the exposed body areas as single lesions. *Leishmania* amastigotes were detected by light microscopy on the Giemsa-stained smears prepared from lesion aspirations, confirming clinical diagnosis.

Furthermore, clinical manifestations suggestive of visceralization of infection were not elicited in these patients. The formol gel test, the only suitable preliminary assay that was available to us during the initial stage, was carried out as a screening test for visceralization of leishmanial infections. None of the cases showed positivity, indicating parasite confinement to the skin,

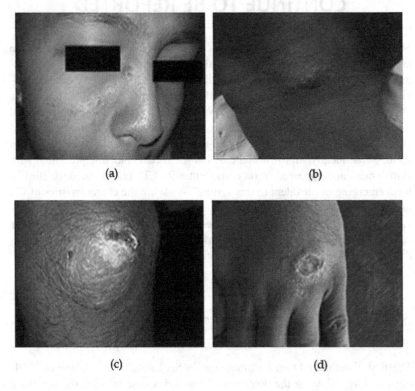

(a)   (b)

(c)   (d)

FIGURE 3.1 Classical developmental stages of CL observed in some locally infected patients. (a) An early papule with an ulcerating nodule. (b) nodule. (c) nodule with central ulceration. and (d) completed ulcer.

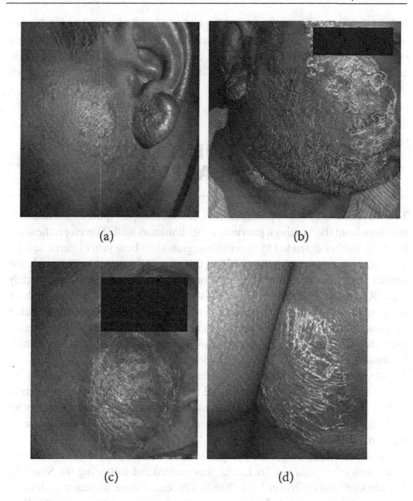

(a)

(b)

(c)

(d)

FIGURE 3.2 Some non-classical manifestations observed in patients with CL in Sri Lanka. (a) Surrounding induration with central ulceration possibly with secondary bacterial infection leading to crusting; (b) extensive lesion with superficial spread with crusting on the lesion and indurated margin; (c) atypical plaque–type lesion in right face; (d): atypical plaque–type lesion in buttock. (Data from Siriwardana Y et al., "Leishmania donovani induced cutaneous leishmaniasis: An insight into atypical clinical variants in Sri Lanka," *Journal of Tropical Medicine* (2019):1–11.)

at least in the few studied cases, though the investigation was not sufficient to exclude concurrent or long-term possibility of visceralization (Siriwardana et al., 2003). A clear majority of these cases were from Northern Sri Lanka, and they were mostly soldiers working in close association with scrub jungles in the North.

3.3 SUBSEQUENT STUDIES ON CLINICAL PROFILE

Towards the end of 2003, patients with CL continued to report in considerable numbers from the Southern province in Sri Lanka as well. Therefore, the studies were further extended to cover this region also. Few years later, a second analysis covered patients reported from this part of the country. This study too further confirmed the clinical profile consistent with CL, at least in the study area (Rajapaksa et al., 2007). In contrast to the previous findings, a Southern Sri Lankan study identified patients from both rural and urban areas within the Southern province. There were higher proportions of younger (10–19 years) individuals, almost equal proportions of males and females, and a bi-annual seasonal variation of case presentation.

It was then apparent that the true case distribution can be wider than initially thought. The studies commenced to include an epidemiological arm as well to study true case burden, spatiotemporal distribution, and risk factors for disease transmission (discussed in subsequent chapters), while surveillance on the clinical profile continued.

A third larger study including 400 cases originating from the North, South and other areas in Sri Lanka was carried out following the Southern Sri Lankan study (Siriwardana, 2008). The cases were screened with more sensitive diagnostic tools including *in vitro* parasite cultivation and/or PCR techniques that had been newly established in the author's institution by that time. This study further confirmed the skin confinement of local leishmanial infections and a clinical profile mainly similar to that described in the first study, except for the wider case distribution within the island. The wider age range group was affected (1–82 years), including both sexes. The majority of patients were soldiers. Majority had evidence to suggest disease acquisition from the same region and less than 1% patients showed nonspecific systemic features. Over 70% of these cases were parasitologically confirmed. Involvement of young adults aged 21–40 years, males, occurrence of single lesions on exposed body areas and belonging to previously described typical lesion stages were observed in this study also. Most (80.2%) of the lesions had been first detected ≤8 months before the case presentation. The main classical stages of lesion development (papules, nodules, ulcerating nodules and completed ulcers) were identified. Papular, nodular, and ulcerative forms were seen in nearly equal proportions. Also, few cases with atypical manifestations were first described in this study (Siriwardana, 2008). The formol gel test was negative in all the patients. With the improved infrastructure, we were able to offer a 2-year free follow-up facility for all diagnosed patients, which later on indicated no signs of visceral involvement (unpublished work of the author).

Multiple studies carried out during the middle part of the epidemic had repeatedly supported the clinical profile of CL. (Rajapaksa et al., 2007; Nawaratna et al., 2007; Samaranayake et al., 2008; Siriwardana et al., 2010, ; Semage et al., 2014; Sandanayaka et al., 2014; Galgamuwa et al., 2017).

3.4 FORWARD JOURNEY

By the end of 2014, CL remained the main clinical entity in Sri Lanka, except for a few sporadic reports on visceral infection that is discussed in the forthcoming chapters. *Leishmania donovani* parasites are generally not known to have animal reservoirs. Early case detection and treatment is considered an important step towards reducing parasite reservoirs. The need for an accurate clinical suspicion in the field as well as hospital setting was identified. Clinical markers that are useful for field screening and clinical decision-making in leishmaniasis were also described for the first time in global literature (Siriwardana et al., 2015). None of the studies showed evidence for visceralization at presentation, during treatment, or during follow-up. But it is known that parasite virulence and epidemiological characteristics can change over time. Therefore, our clinical surveillance was continued as an essential step. Though the majority of initial cases were from Northern areas in Sri Lanka, the Southern province contributed the major proportion of cutaneous leishmaniasis (CL) reported during later stages, probably due to the availability of services of a dermatologist for the region, improved degree of awareness, and convenient transport systems between patient areas and the Central laboratory in Colombo.

Though self-cure or cure with treatment are the accepted norms in skin infections of CL, achieving a total parasite clearance is known to be difficult in leishmaniasis. The remaining dormant parasites can give rise to full-blown leishmaniasis or recurrence at later stages. With the identification of *L. donovani* as the cause of CL in Sri Lanka, the possibility of visceralization of currently dermotropic strains and emergence of other clinical forms or concurrent mucosal leishmaniasis (ML) and VL with CL could not be disregarded. Therefore, continued efforts to raise awareness, patient diagnostic facilities, and continued surveillance were also required during this time.

Other Clinical Forms Emerge in Sri Lanka

4

4.1 POSSIBILITY OF VISCERAL AND MUCOSAL INFECTIONS

In spite of the growing number of cases of cutaneous leishmaniasis, the genetically distinct nature and the original visceralizing nature of the causative species provided justification for consideration of the presence or subsequent emergence of other potentially dangerous mucosal and visceral clinical forms of leishmaniasis in Sri Lanka. In order to detect such occurrences, it was necessary to make the clinicians aware of the purely laboratory-based local information. Diagnostic facilities to include bone marrow examination procedures for patients with suspected visceral leishmaniasis were established in the Department of Parasitology in the Faculty of Medicine of the University of Colombo (UCFM) in 2005. Our first attempt was a discussion carried out by myself with a few interested physicians at the National Hospital in Colombo to watch out for possible cases of visceral leishmaniasis. As a result, a young female from Northern Sri Lanka who presented with pyrexia of unknown origin (PUO) of 6 month duration was investigated by bone marrow examination for *Leishmania* spp. This revealed the presence of *Leishmania* parasites. This was the first confirmation of clinical visceral leishmaniasis in our laboratory. This patient was successfully treated with sodium stibogluconate (SSG). The case had been followed up for 12 years and reported only recently after adequate follow-up data to exclude the possibility of relapse or other sequelae (Siriwardana et al., 2017). The patient did not show any complication of leishmaniasis and remains apparently disease-free at the time of writing this book.

DOI: 10.1201/9781003281801-4

During the same year, two patients with oral lesions were also reported, and the authors have attributed these to mucosal tissue localization of leishmaniasis (Rajapaksa et al., 2005). Case number 1 was a soldier from Omanthai, a location in Northern Sri Lanka. Case 2 was a school child from Ambalantota, a location in Southern Sri Lanka. Both had lesions over the inner side of the lower lip. Diagnosis was confirmed by microscopy on lesion material. Both patients had responded well to standard anti-leishmanial treatment with SSG (Rajapaksa et al., 2005). No follow-up data are available on these cases.

Possibility of direct, lymphatic, or hematogenous spread of parasites from an adjacent bite site on the face or even a distant skin site should be considered in these two cases as it is very unlikely for a primary lesion to occur after a sandfly bite of the identified sites of infection. Also, the inner side of the lower lip contains modified cutaneous tissue and not true mucosa. Therefore, these two cases could have ideally been categorized as spread of cutaneous infection to involve lip skin. Occurrence of true mucosal leishmaniasis is uncertain in these two cases. However, these two reports paved the way for raised vigilance among us to look in to mucotropism of leishmaniasis as well.

Following this report, a third case of locally transmitted true mucosal leishmaniasis was reported in 2010 in a 52-year-old man from Mahiyangana in the Central province in Sri Lanka (Rathnayake et al., 2010). This patient initially had a small discoloured patch on the face near the angle of his mouth which was negative for leishmaniasis by light microscopic examination of lesion scrapings. Further investigations on leishmaniasis had not been carried out until 6 years later when he presented to us with severe mucosal tissue destruction. The upper lips were swollen and posterior part of the soft palate and nasal septum were severely damaged, leaving large deficiencies. Diagnosis of mucosal leishmaniasis was confirmed by examination of mucosal lesion tissue scrapings by microscopy and PCR. The patient had inherent immune deficiency and co-infection with extra pulmonary tuberculosis. The patient responded well for anti-leishmanial treatment with sodium stibogluconate (SSG). His destructive lesions were well-confined to the mucosal tissue. There was no facial involvement or signs of facial inflammation. This enables us to conclude this as true mucosal leishmaniasis.

Meanwhile, another reported case of locally acquired visceral leishmaniasis was available in 2007 from Northern Sri Lanka (Abeygunasekara et al., 2007). The patient did not have a history of fever. There had been massive hepatosplenomegaly, anaemia (7.9 g/dL), reduced WBC count (3.6×10^9/L), elevated ESR (160 mm in 1st hour), raised serum globulin levels, and reactive hyperplasia of all cell lines in bone marrow. Based on these findings, the patient was clinically diagnosed to have a lymphoma. Subsequently, *Leishmania* spp.

parasites had been demonstrated in both liver Kupffer cells and in bone marrow histiocytes. Unfortunately, no treatment or follow-up data are available on this case.

Few years later in 2011, occurrence of indigenous visceral leishmaniasis was confirmed in a 57-year-old male from Vavuniya district in Northern Sri Lanka who presented with pyrexia of unknown origin of 6-month duration (Ranasinghe et al., 2012). There was an occupational history of working in the jungle in Vavuniya district in Northern Sri Lanka as a soldier for several months during the period of political unrest, immediately prior to the occurrence of symptoms. Diagnosis had been confirmed by microscopy and *in vitro* cultivation of *Leishmania spp.* in bone marrow. Case management or follow-up details are not available on this patient as well.

The same report had included details of the causative species of visceral leishmaniasis in this patient (Ranasinghe et al., 2012). The parasite had been identified as *Leishmania donovani* MON-37, the same organism responsible for skin infections, though this was not backed up by true genetic-based studies.

4.2 RECENT CASES AND TRENDS

Patients suspected of having visceral leishmaniasis (n = 120) fulfilling at least two of six criteria (fever >2 weeks, weight loss, tiredness affecting daily functions, splenomegaly, hepatomegaly, and anemia) were studied using clinico-epidemiological, immunological, and haematological parameters in our network for active surveillance of visceral leishmaniasis. Few more cases of visceral leishmaniasis were detected during the subsequent years through this activity. The first formal records on follow-up of visceral leishmaniasis patients were made available in this study (Siriwardana et al., 2017). This report described seven cases; four progressive treated cases (group A) and three nonprogressive, potentially asymptomatic, and observed only (group B) cases. Clinical cases were treated with systemic sodium stibogluconate, amphotericin B, or miltefosine, and all patients were followed up at the leishmaniasis clinic of the University of Colombo for 3 years, with the 2005 case followed up for 9 years (and 15 years as at present).

All treated cases have responded well to anti-leishmanial treatment without relapses up to the time of writing of this book, except for one patient who died due to a nonrelated cause. Clinical features subsided in all nonprogressive cases and did not develop suggestive clinical features or changes in laboratory parameters. Nonprogressive cases could be asymptomatic cases of leishmanial infection. Reported cases have been originated from different districts within

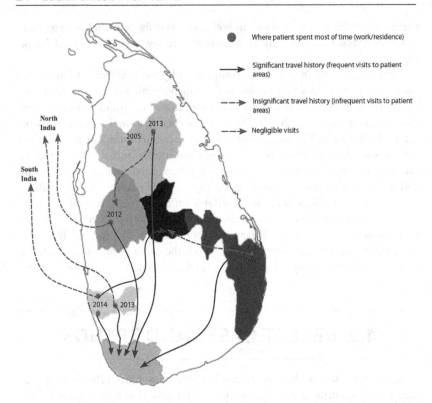

FIGURE 4.1 Temporal distribution of residences and likely place of infection acquisition of VL cases in Sri Lanka over space. (Data from Siriwardana et al., "Emergence of visceral leishmaniasis in Sri Lanka: A newly established Health Threat" *Pathogens and Global Health.* 111(6) (2017):317–26.)

the country. Majority had a travel history to identified local foci of cutaneous leishmaniasis (Figure 4.1). Approximate incubation time was highly variable in these patients (3 months to many years) (Siriwardana et al., 2017). Approximate time taken from first appearance/suspicion of one or more clinical features to the point of laboratory diagnosis was also highly variable (3 months–6 years). None of these patients had a past history of cutaneous leishmaniasis, suggestive skin lesions, or manifestations suggestive of PKDL. However, one patient had a macular, generalized skin rash which resolved spontaneously during anti-leishmanial therapy.

Hairy cell leukaemia, typhoid fever, lymphoma, and diabetes were identified as coexisting illnesses in four of seven patients. However, it was not clear whether these conditions preceded or followed leishmanial infections (Figure 4.2).

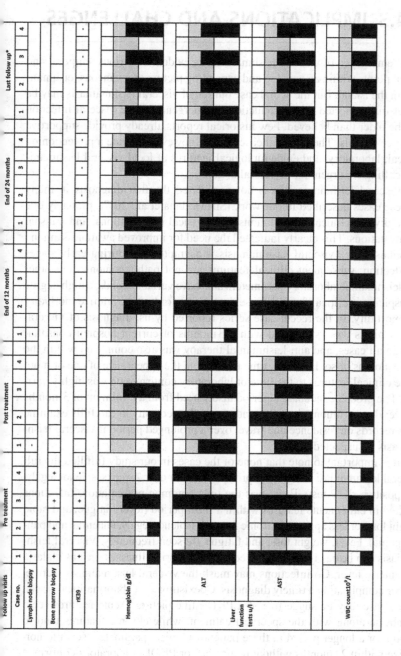

FIGURE 4.2 Laboratory profile and trends of clinically progressive and treated individuals. (Data from Siriwardana et al., "Emergence of visceral leishmaniasis in Sri Lanka: A newly established Health Threat" *Pathogens and Global Health.* 111(6) (2017):317–26.)

4.3 IMPLICATIONS AND CHALLENGES

Local emergence of visceral leishmaniasis is evident at various temporal and spatial points within an existing and expanding picture of cutaneous leishmaniasis in the island. But the actual case burden of visceral leishmaniasis may be higher than reported and introduction or emergence of the visceral infection may be older than believed. Few historical reports already provide supportive evidence for this. The detected cases so far, however, provide a projection on clinical, laboratory, and epidemiological features of local visceral leishmaniasis, calling for urgent multisectoral action.

Visceral leishmaniasis was not considered the first diagnosis in many of these cases described in our work (Siriwardana et al., 2017), probably due to the diverse clinical presentations, nonclassical combinations, and unusual manifestations. This clearly indicated the need for improved awareness among clinicians. Since visceral leishmaniasis is asymptomatic during early stages of infection, subsequent clinical features are not pathognomonic and other non-leishmanial laboratory parameters also have variable trends; a high degree of suspicion is critical for early case detection in order to minimize morbidity and mortality. In the recent case series reported by us, diagnosis of visceral leishmaniasis was established within 3 months of current hospital consultations in all cases, and anti-leishmanial therapy was also completed within the next 3 months or so. However, time taken from the appearance of one or more of the clinical features to the time of laboratory confirmation was highly variable. The probable incubation period also varied from a minimum of 3 months to several years among the cases, indicating the necessity to carefully examine one's records on residence and travel over a prolonged period if visceral leishmaniasis is suspected.

It is important to note that none of the cases in our study fulfilled the full visceral leishmaniasis diagnostic profile (fever for over 2 weeks, splenomegaly, and positive rK39 test). Fever was the only common presentation. Infections resulted in either acute features within a short period (fever, fatigue, and rapid weight loss) or less apparent chronic features (splenomegaly, anaemia, and pancytopenia). Fever, weight loss, and fatigue are seen frequently. Visceral leishmaniasis can be easily misdiagnosed as other febrile illnesses such as malaria and enteric fever. Co-infections may mask the visceral leishmaniasis picture, further complicating a timely diagnosis. Coexisting skin abnormalities as seen in one case may be suggestive of a PKDL-like picture. Acute features seem to subside along with the specific treatment, while chronic features tend to remain for a longer period in these patients. Clinical parameters seem to normalize within 24 months without recurrence or PKDL. Laboratory-confirmed infections with nonprogressive clinical disease point towards the important questions such as whether they are self-resolving minor leishmanial infections or whether concurrent accidental detection of still subclinical or asymptomatic infection during investigations for another illness that shares similar clinical features with visceral leishmaniasis.

Though only a proportion of cutaneous leishmaniasis cases are offered pretreatment laboratory confirmation due to practical difficulties in the local setting, suspected visceral leishmaniasis always require pretreatment confirmation. Sero-conversion in local cutaneous leishmaniasis is being currently investigated (Siriwardana et al., 2018). Negative rK39 results of two out of four local visceral leishmaniasis cases indicate the lack of sensitivity/reliability of this assay in Sri Lankan patients, possibly due to the antigenic differences in local parasites as compared to traditionally visceralizing *L. donovani*. The current findings, therefore, stress the need for more locally appropriate serological tools. In spite of this, sero-positivity had been demonstrated in endemic but apparently healthy inhabitants (rK39 assay positivity in some apparently healthy individuals, data unpublished), indicating possible sero-conversion without disease, self-resolved past infection, or asymptomatic visceral leishmaniasis.

Most local infections responded well to the anti-leishmanials with no apparent evidence of recurrence, though it might be too early to make generalized conclusions based on small samples. Neighbouring India reports resistance to first-line anti-leishmanials and often uses second-line drugs such as amphotericin B. Expensive and toxic anti-leishmanial usage may cause a huge economic burden and serious side effects on patients. Sri Lankans are frequent travellers to Bihar in India and African countries where visceral leishmaniasis is endemic for religious or employment purposes. Management protocols and treatment response patterns of visceral leishmaniasis show great variability within different global endemic settings. Local anti-visceral leishmaniasis therapy has multiple options so far (Siriwardana et al., 2018). The current global trend is to treat clinical illness and closely follow up asymptomatic cases owing to the toxicity and complexity of available anti-leishmanials (WHO, 2010). Evidence-based revisit to local protocols may be necessary in future. All cases are likely to have acquired the infection locally, although overseas travel history was present in two cases. Local infections appear to be responsive to the first-line antimonials which is encouraging when there is *L. donovani*–associated drug resistance in other settings (Mohapatra, 2014).

Majority of reported cases so far pointed towards a history of travel to/stay in known cutaneous leishmaniasis areas in Southern or Northern Sri Lanka. Two independent foci of disease transmission in North and South (Siriwardana et al., 2010; Siriwardana et al., 2019) and case clustering (Kariyawasam et al., 2015) have been suggested by previous studies. But, none of the reported visceral leishmaniasis patients, except two, were residents of these areas. One of them spent most of his time in Northern Sri Lanka over the preceding 9 years, and the other patient's residence was in South. No other cases of visceral leishmaniasis have been reported from these foci. Low index of suspicion among clinicians and cross immunity resulting from prevailing cutaneous leishmaniasis strains (Zhang et al., 2014) might be contributing factors for this.

Spontaneous remission of visceral leishmaniasis has been reported rarely (Mouri et al., 2015). In this back drop, high degree of clinical suspicion and investigations are necessary to detect any possible case, which might act as a parasite reservoir to the community.

Establishment of visceral leishmaniasis can result in considerable socio-economic ill effects in the country, in addition to the increased mortality and high health cost in management. Wide prevalence of incriminated vector species (*Phlebotomus argentipes*), free movement and possible intermingling of non-immune and immune populations, silent nature of initial infections, poor awareness on visceral leishmaniasis, and scarcity of scientific information may viciously facilitate delayed intervention and silent disease progression. With increased air travel, particularly to neighbouring India, there is a risk of imported leishmaniasis too. Local transmission cycle is likely to be receptive to the foreign parasite strains, facilitating the spread of the disease.

4.4 ASYMPTOMATIC
L. DONOVANI INFECTION

Few countries in the SEA region aimed at elimination of visceral leishmaniasis initially by 2015 in which multiple difficulties were encountered at the commencement and during the progression of the activities (Chowdhury et al., 2014; Gurunath et al., 2014; Bhandari et al., 2011). Among many challenges, the fact that only a minority of *L. donovani* infections progress to clinical disease was identified as a leading cause. Various studies have described asymptomatic infection in different ways that include subclinical forms in serologically positive individuals and minimal or self-resolving infection or laboratory positivity without clinical features (Badaro et al., 1986; Srivastava et al., 2013). Asymptomatic carriers are known to play an important role in maintaining the disease/infection epidemic in a community (Stauch et al., 2011). Asymptomatic individuals are not identified or treated in many communities, and the treatment with expensive and toxic drugs is not justified even if the infection status is confirmed. However, the role of such infections may be important in the society, indicating the need for treatment. Therefore, careful understanding of the problem is important with regard to prevention and control of leishmaniasis in a given setting. Different endemic settings have described the asymptomatic: clinical disease ratio in *L. donovani/Leishmania infantum*. Variable figures have been observed in the Indian sub-continent (Stauch et al., 2011; Ostyn et al., 2011).

4.5 CHALLENGES POSED BY ASYMPTOMATIC INFECTIONS

Identification of risk factors for infection, determinants of disease progression, and clinical and diagnostic markers for early detection of asymptomatic infections remain the three main challenges at present. Prognosis of asymptomatic infection at the individual level has not yet been fully studied. Such drawbacks might also prevent utilizing an opportunity for early intervention.

Progression and outcome of *L. donovani* infection may possibly be the interaction between host, parasite, and the environmental factors. Various associations including genetic factors (Mohamed et al., 2004), malnutrition (Cerf et al., 1987), infection in family members or the neighbours (Mary et al., 1992), and poor housing conditions (Custodio et al., 2012; Bern et al., 2000) have been identified as risk factors. In neighbouring India, genetic associations have also been reported (Mehrotra et al., 2011). Conflicting results have been obtained with regard to ownership of animals, (Bern et al., 2000) and use of bed-nets (Picado et al., 2010). There are no widely validated markers for asymptomatic *L. donovani* infection. Diagnostic assays are also directed at identifying clinical disease in cutaneous leishmaniasis and visceral leishmaniasis. These studies have demonstrated that some infected individuals tend to develop an effective immune response without clinical disease. Immunological indicators (Sundar et al., 2002, 2006; Vallur et al., 2016) and sensitive molecular biological tools (Silva et al., 2013; Sudarshan et al., 2014) seem to be important in detecting such infections. There had been associations between sero-prevalence and age (Siriwardana et al., 2018) and extent of sero-conversion and progression to clinical visceral leishmaniasis (Hasker et al., 2014). The ability of asymptomatic persons to infect sandfly vectors is another aspect which requires a better understanding. Detailed entomological studies on the vector's behaviour and methods such as sand fly saliva antibody tests (Clements et al., 2010) may be invaluable in this.

In Sri Lanka, the extent of asymptomatic infection is not yet fully known. Few cases of visceral leishmaniasis reported by us recently already point towards asymptomatic infection and self-resolving infection (Siriwardana et al., 2017). Asymptomatic infection has posed a huge challenge to the clinician in initial suspicion and to the scientist in convincing the curative sector with regard to the necessity of early suspicion in patients with self-resolving febrile illness.

However, at present, it is not possible to predict which asymptomatic individual will develop clinical visceral disease. Risk factors for infection and prognosis are also not fully understood. Four patients with only sero-positivity and four patients with parasite positivity are being followed up at present. Sero-conversion of dermotropic *L. donovani* in Sri Lanka has been demonstrated in some patients recently (Siriwardana et al., 2018). Attempts to identify clinical and molecular biological markers for asymptomatic infection, risk factors, and predictors of prognosis would be of great value in this setting.

Changing Trends in Cutaneous Leishmaniasis

5

5.1 CHANGING TRENDS IN CLASSICAL MANIFESTATIONS

In 2017, trends of cutaneous leishmaniasis (CL) during a period of 14 years (2001–2013) was studied in a large set of patients representing early, middle, and late stages of the epidemic (Siriwardana et al., 2019). Though a previously described broad profile of cutaneous leishmaniasis still remains applicable and undisturbed, it was interesting to note the time-dependent changing patterns within this main profile. This study showed changing patterns and constant patterns of different clinical and socio-demographic features. It is known that the parasitological and epidemiological characteristics can demonstrate changing trends during progression of an epidemic of leishmaniasis (Amin et al., 2013).

CL seems to occur mainly in young adult males as single lesions on exposed body areas without evidence of visceralization (Siriwardana et al., 2017). The clinical profile was not gender- or age-dependent. However, it was interesting to note the increasing involvement of females and elderly individuals (>40 years) over time, in spite of unchanged broad clinical picture of CL. Older individuals reported increasing proportions of early and ulcerated lesions over time as compared to younger individuals (Siriwardana et al., 2019). Spatial distribution of cases of cutaneous leishmaniasis had expanded

DOI: 10.1201/9781003281801-5

since the onset of the epidemic. However, bi-annual seasonal variation of case presentation with two peaks corresponding to monsoon rainfall patterns in the country was observed since early stages and remained constant during subsequent years.

These findings formed a rational background to conclude that cutaneous leishmaniasis still remain the main clinical entity in Sri Lanka. Its clinical profile also remains rather constant, with minor changes occurring within the main profile, while other clinical forms of leishmaniasis emerge. Though trends of major changes are not observed within the profile of cutaneous leishmaniasis, these minor and continued clinical and socio-demographic changes point towards peri-domestication of the transmission cycles, increased host immunity, spatial expansion, or changing socio-demographic patterns. It is important to carry out periodic surveillance of the clinical and epidemiological characteristics and case presentation characteristics in the study population to further understand the changing trends within the existing picture. Main disease foci are still reported in resource-limited areas in the local setting. A reduction in self-referral time was seen, though there were some chronic lesions identified during the late stages. Accurate clinical suspicion especially in a laboratory resource–limited setting is required to enhance case detection in new disease foci.

5.2 ATYPICAL CUTANEOUS MANIFESTATIONS

A recent study reported a prevalence of 13% for atypical manifestations associated with cutaneous leishmaniasis in Sri Lanka (AtCL) and identified this category as a different clinical entity (Siriwardana et al., 2019). These lesions did not show age or gender association. Majority of AtCL lesions were single and had a typical onset. However, AtCL showed a low parasite positivity rate as compared to classical cutaneous leishmaniasis infections. Half of the early lesions that demonstrated a non-classical onset (lesion other than painless acne form papules over the skin) developed in to AtCL later on as well. The study also showed that AtCL was more frequently seen in Northern Sri Lanka as compared to other regions (Figure 5.1). Also., residents of other regions visiting Northern parts of the island and acquiring infection there developed higher proportions of AtCL as compared to residents in North (60.9% vs 30.6%). Atypical lesions were associated with a delayed response to standard anti-leishmanial treatment when compared with classical lesions.

Atypical manifestations in cutaneous leishmaniasis comprise an important category that can complicate initial clinical screening in an endemic

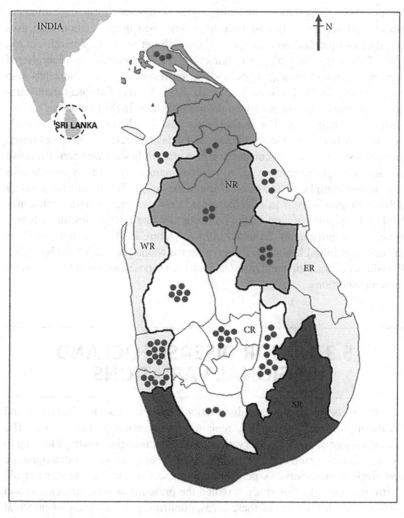

NR- Northern region
SR- Southern region
CR- Central region
WR- Western region
ER- Eastern region

— - Administrative margins of regions
— - Administrative margins of districts

FIGURE 5.1 Geographical locations of cases of atypical cutaneous leishmaniasis in Sri Lanka. (Siriwardana Y et al., "Leishmania donovani induced cutaneous leishmaniasis: An insight into atypical clinical variants in Sri Lanka," *Journal of Tropical Medicine* (2019):1–11.)

setting. Many clinical forms including erysepeloid, zosteriform, disseminated, lupoid, and verrucous lesions have been described in association with usually dermotropic *Leishmania* species (Carvalho et al., 2017; Meireles et al., 2017; Tomasini et al., 2017; Iftikhar et al., 2003). Genetic variation altered immune pathological sequences, and varied response to treatment has also been reported in AtCL (Guimaraes et al., 2016). Entity of atypical manifestations seen among cutaneous leishmaniasis infections in Sri Lanka may constitute an important group. The non-ulcerative and non-disturbing nature of early skin lesions in classical leishmaniasis can delay self-referral. Atypical onset, unusual lesion features, occurrence on proximal body sites, and non-ulcerative course and high prevalence of in non-leishmanial areas in atypical lesions can further complicate the clinical diagnosis by leading to misdiagnosis or delayed diagnosis even in referred cases. Low parasite positivity rates may further delay point-of-care diagnosis using first-line microscopy and a timely laboratory confirmation. Eventual clinical picture in AtCL is dependent on the nature of initial lesion, location within the country, and affected body site. Parasite strain variation and host factors were proposed as possible reasons for these observations.

5.3 MAJOR DISEASE FOCI AND REGIONAL VARIATIONS

In spite of the widening case distribution within the country, Northern and Southern provinces continued to remain as main patient prevalent areas. The author's informal clinical observations and epidemiological findings leading to further study reported in year 2019examined the long-term socio-demographic and clinical characteristics pertaining to these two foci (Siriwardana et al., 2010). Interestingly, this study revealed the presence of two independent and different profiles in each of these areas, confirming the accuracy of informal observations.

Patients presenting from different geographical locations for laboratory confirmation at the department of Parasitology, Faculty of Medicine in the University of Colombo for cutaneous leishmaniasis over a period of 14 years (2001–2013) were studied. A sample of 600 patients (first 200 each from the early (2001–2003), mid (2004–2009), and late (2009–2013) stages of the epidemic) was identified. Majority of patients presented from North and South. They had acquired the infection from the same region (data not shown). A similar pattern had been shown during the early stages of the epidemic also. Both foci demonstrated a bi-annual seasonal variation in case presentation.

Two peaks were observed during the early and later parts of the year. This was observed since early stages of the epidemic. Studies on different subsets of patients have made similar observations with association of environmental factors (temperature, wind speed, and humidity) as contributing factors for disease transmission (Galgamuwa et al., 2018).

Though the majority of patients were males in both foci, the proportion of affected females in the Southern focus (SF) was clearly higher than that of the Northern focus (NF). All age groups were almost equally affected in the South, while young adults were mainly affected in the North. Lesions identified in the Southern study presented early (78.6% vs 62.2% in NF). In spite of this, the proportion of ulcerative stages was clearly high in SF (52.5% vs 30% in the North), while the mean duration of a lesion was also less (5.62 vs 10.7 months), and proportion of large lesions was also higher in SF (47% vs 32%, >2 cm) as than the same reported at NF (10.7 months).

Lesions observed in the South were also more likely to be erythematous or hypopigmented as compared to those in the North. Their edges were less regular. Nodular lesions in the South were more likely to have surface squamation, and ulcerative lesions were less dry in NF. The surrounding skin of lesions in the South also showed a higher degree of skin scaling, skin inflammation, or pigmentation changes as compared to those reported at the Northern study site.

There were a small number of patients presenting from the Western focus or the districts in the Western Central and North-Western regions. Patients presenting from North-Western and Central foci showed consistency with the features reported in the North (Figure 5.2), while patients presenting from the Western focus had a mixed picture.

Gender- and age-based analyses were carried out for the two sites to assess the age and sex dependency of clinical characteristics.

From these findings, it was evident that skin lesions reported in the South were more likely to present early, had a lower mean duration, were enlarged in size, and show early ulceration rather than having a tendency to multiply, while leishmanial skin lesion in the North remained smaller and had a higher mean lesion duration and a comparatively higher proportion, showing late multiplication and late ulceration. Lesions at the Southern focus were more inflammatory as indicated by a higher proportion of lesions showing surface scaling during nodular stages and lesion and skin inflammatory changes as compared to those reported at the Northern focus, which were less inflammatory. Rapid progression seen in the South may indicate a more pronounced host reaction, or parasite strains found in the North may be less likely to exert a host reaction but progress as better survivors within the host.

These findings led us to conclude that there are two slightly different profiles in each site with differences in the rate of disease progression. The Northern focus showed a relatively slow progression, while infections in the

Southern focus were more prone to show rapid ulceration and enlargement of lesions. These differences were identified from early stages of the epidemic. Consistency of each clinical pattern over time in its spatial location further favoured the hypothesis for long-term existence of stabilized and independent disease transmission in these areas (Siriwardana et al., 2019).

A more recent study included military persons serving Northern Sri Lanka. Authors have analysed the clinical profile of cutaneous leishmaniasis. Their findings were consistent with previously described findings in the North. Soldiers serving Northern Sri Lanka are residents of different parts of the country. Therefore, these findings also point towards a parasitic aetiology and not a host association for the observed clinical outcomes (Gunathilaka et al., 2020).

5.4 OTHER LOCATIONS

The study further indicated that other case-reporting areas in North-Western and Central foci possess many characteristics similar to those of Northern focus. They are likely to have acquired the spreading infection from the Northern focus. The Western province had a mixed picture (Figure 5.2). This area is a highly commercial, urban, and a highly populated area in the country, with the commercial capital as the central point, and it is not known to be a leishmaniasis-prevalent area. Sandfly vectors of leishmaniasis are widely prevalent in the country, including the Western province. Therefore, reported cases were probably due to increased patient travel between Western province and disease prevalent areas.

5.5 COURSE OF SKIN LESIONS

A subsequent analysis revealed the presence of two different lesion patterns in each geographical location (Siriwardana et al., 2021). However, they were not confined to these regions. Therefore, it was necessary to further study the true clinical differences that are independent of geo-locations.

A description of the different lesion types identified within the profile of cutaneous leishmaniasis was available recently (Siriwardana et al., 2019). A total of 550 patients with parasitological-confirmed classical cutaneous leishmaniasis were examined in this study. Nearly 1/3 of early lesions (<3 months

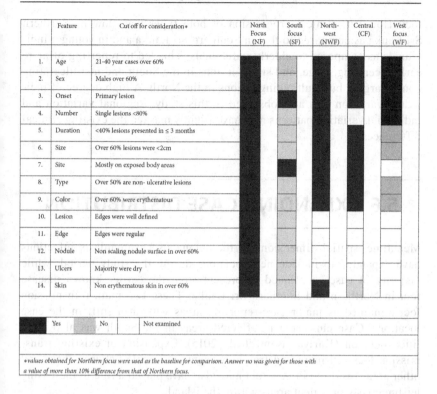

	Feature	Cut off for consideration*	North Focus (NF)	South focus (SF)	North-west (NWF)	Central (CF)	West focus (WF)
1.	Age	21-40 year cases over 60%					
2.	Sex	Males over 60%					
3.	Onset	Primary lesion					
4.	Number	Single lesions <80%					
5.	Duration	<40% lesions presented in ≤ 3 months					
6.	Size	Over 60% lesions were <2cm					
7.	Site	Mostly on exposed body areas					
8.	Type	Over 50% are non- ulcerative lesions					
9.	Color	Over 60% were erythematous					
10.	Lesion	Edges were well defined					
11.	Edge	Edges were regular					
12.	Nodule	Non scaling nodule surface in over 60%					
13.	Ulcers	Majority were dry					
14.	Skin	Non erythematous skin in over 60%					

	Yes		No		Not examined		

*values obtained for Northern focus were used as the baseline for comparison. Answer no was given for those with a value of more than 10% difference from that of Northern focus.

FIGURE 5.2 Relationship of different clinical compositions to geographical locations of *L. donovani* skin infection in Sri Lanka. (Siriwardana Y, Deepachandi B, Weliange Sde, Udagedara C, Wickremarathne C, Warnasuriya W, et al. First evidence for two independent and different leishmaniasis transmission foci in Sri Lanka: Recent introduction or long-term existence? *Journal of Tropical Medicine* (2019):1–11.)

duration) showed enlargement (>2 cm), while ulceration was also observed in nearly half of them. The proportion of enlarged lesions remained constant over time. However, among the chronic (>12 months duration) lesions, half remained small (<2 cm in size) and nearly 1/4 remained as non-ulcerated non-enlarged papules. Late non-ulcerative types, NUTs, showed a higher tendency to multiply while remaining small (<2 cm diameter). All types of lesions progressed through classical stages described in lesion development in leishmaniasis. None had systemic manifestations or primary clinical evidence of visceralization.

Two lesion types (early ulcerative type or UTs and non-ulcerative type: NUTs) were described based on these observations. Lesion types were independent of the geographical location. Both types were reported in both foci. However, clinical progression of both types was slow in Northern Sri Lanka as compared to that in Southern Sri Lanka and in younger individuals as compared to elderly individuals. This led to reporting of more early ulcerating, large, and single lesions in the South and non-ulcerating non-enlarging but multiplying lesions in the North. A high degree of individual variation was also observed in this study. Regional variation and individual variation patterns may have slightly masked the existing clinical differences.

5.6 EXPANDING CASE DISTRIBUTION

Meantime, spatial dimensions of the cutaneous leishmaniasis infections have expanded to include new locations during the study period, while majority of cases continued to present from the earlier known disease foci in Northern and Southern Sri Lanka. These two main transmission foci remained as major case-reporting areas without a shift in the case locations. Case clustering in affected areas in the South was also identified later on (Kariyawasam et al., 2015). Expansion of existing transmission foci and increased free movements of people between these and other areas resulting in new foci may also have played a role in increasing leishmaniasis-prevalent areas within the island.

Improved awareness among clinicians and availability of a decentralized facility for microscopic diagnosis at hospitals may have facilitated initial screening and laboratory confirmation of cases. Seasonal variation patterns of case distribution are useful in timing vector control activities.

Cutaneous leishmaniasis seems to affect a wider age range (1–81 years, data not shown) and both genders with male preponderance since the onset of the epidemic. Though this male preponderance still remains unchanged, a changing age–sex pattern with increased involvement of older age groups and females during the later stages may be indicative of an association with behavioural patterns and peri-domestication that increases the risk of disease being transmitted to them. However, there is a considerable proportion of lesions that were either presented or detected later than a year from the onset/notice of the skin lesion, indicating the need for improved self-referrals and case suspicion. Increase in the number of single and early lesions may be indicative of better awareness and case detection rates, though this may also be due to rapid progression of skin lesions which need to be confirmed by other means.

5.7 IMPLICATIONS FOR PRACTICE

Main clinical forms of leishmaniasis are known to be species-specific to a large extent. However, detection of all three clinical forms of leishmaniasis, evidence for long-term existence of them in the country, expansion of case distribution in cutaneous form, and changing trends in clinical profiles together with a genetically distinct parasite species in Sri Lanka set a typical example for a mismatch between the causative species and its outcome. Already observed unusual sequelae are many. These unforeseen outcomes cannot be disregarded. Identification of these sequelae and an understanding on the underlying mechanisms are necessary to achieve successful disease control (Zhang et al., 2014). High serological response was also reported among cutaneous leishmaniasis patients in Sri Lanka. This, however, is indicative of a potential for visceralization, though it requires further confirmation and in-depth analysis *(discussed in subsequent chapters)* (Siriwardana et al., 2018). Possible outcomes of leishmaniasis in this country cannot be assumed based on what is known for similar settings elsewhere. Local sequelae can take a different route.

In summary, leishmanial infections in Sri Lanka have increasingly shown a widening of spatial distribution in the island during the subsequent years (Siriwardana et al., 2010, 2015). VL and muco-cutaneous leishmaniasis have been reported among few (Rathnayake et al., 2010; Siriwardana et al., 2017), while cutaneous leishmaniasis infections have demonstrated a humoral response, though the extent of visceralization has not yet been fully understood (Siriwardana et al., 2018). Meanwhile, poor treatment response *(discussed in subsequent chapters)* had also been a concern (Refai et al., 2016). Co-infection with other rare and chronic diseases has been reported (Kahandawaaracchchi et al., 2017). All these observations have already established a strong justification for continued clinical surveillance within the country, preferably backed up by parasitological and immunological aspects as well. Full characterization of the clinical profile of such infection can not only aid case detection and management but also help avoid unnecessary treatment costs and side effects and aid the patient-based and community-based interventions for disease control. Attempts on case detection are further discussed in the later chapters of this book.

The Mismatched Parasite

6

The results of the Colombo study together with the work described by others lead to the definitive conclusion that Sri Lankan cutaneous leishmaniasis is caused by *Leishmania donovani*. This has been confirmed by several independent methods as described in the previous sections (MLEE, 6PGDH sequences, micro satellites, cytochrome b, and A2 gene). The local dermotropic parasite was identified as a genetic variant of *Leishmania donovani* (Siriwardana et al., 2007). This finding is of higher significance, with many important implications for patient management and epidemiology of disease, especially in the ongoing increase in reported case numbers.

6.1 STRAIN VARIATION?

Strain variation within *L. donovani* and its dependency on geographical location are already-observed phenomena in the world (Lukes et al., 2007; Zemanova et al., 2004; Kuhls et al., 2005; Mauricio et al., 2001, 2004). New foci of cutaneous leishmaniasis apparently caused by *L. donovani* also continue to be reported in various parts of Africa (Johnson et al., 1993; Elamin et al., 2008) and Asia (Hanly et al., 1998; Sharma et al., 2005; Toz et al., 2009). During the last few years, atypical clinical presentations of the dermotropic *L. donovani* have also been reported, further complicating the understanding of the characteristics of these foci (Flaig et al., 2007; Elamin et al., 2008; Faber et al., 2009). Some studies on *L. donovani* causing cutaneous leishmaniasis have shown genetic similarities to both *L. donovani* and *L. infantum*, the two sibling species that are described within the *L. donovani* complex (Sharma et al., 2005). Other co-existing genetic differences may be numerous and may remain unknown. Two important concerns at this point are the underlying reasons for dermotropism and possible clinical and epidemiological implications arising from them.

6.2 WHY DO NOT THEY VISCERALIZE?

Genetic comparison studies of (CL and VL) cutaneous and visceral leishmaniasis isolates of Sri Lankan origin employing a limited number of samples has provided an insight in to this (Zhang et al., 2014). The study showed that a single cutaneous leishmaniasis isolate examined in the study was severely attenuated in copy numbers of the A2 gene and expression level of A2 proteins when compared to that of a single local visceral leishmaniasis isolate. A2 is considered essential for survival of *Leishmania* in visceral organs. This attenuation was thought to have caused skin confinement of the infection in mice. This study identified two potential genetic variations responsible for the phenotypic differences.

Studies conducted by some of us recently observed a phenotypic association with genetic differences of local *L. donovani* parasites (cutaneous strains, visceralizing strains, and poor responders to treatment). Furthermore, this study revealed a high degree of haplotype variability within the Sri Lankan *Leishmania* parasites. Also, long-term follow-up studies have failed to demonstrate any possibility for visceralization of initial cutaneous leishmaniasis infections at least during first 4 years following detection (Kariyawasam et al., 2017).

Clinical and epidemiological studies also indicate the possible presence of multiple genetic variants within the group of Sri Lankan *Leishmania donovani sensu lato*. Identification of a clearly different clinical entity of atypical lesions within the cutaneous leishmaniasis profile (Siriwardana et al., 2019), primary clinical evidence indicating the presence of two different clinical profiles in Northern and Southern Sri Lanka (Siriwardana et al., 2019), and probably two different clinical types (Siriwardana et al 2021) further support this hypothesis. Host immune status, nutritional status, other genetic factors, and sandfly behaviours may also play a role in the final clinical outcome in this setting.

Findings of phylogenetic studies are dependent on the genetic loci examined in the study (Shaw, 2007). They identify the differences of the genetic loci under study, irrespective of whether these differences reflect the true phenotypic or other functional differences related to pathology (McCall et al., 2013). The complete study of a full genome of *Leishmania* is a very expensive undertaking that requires many other resources. Inclusion of a larger number of genetic loci and a more representative nationwide sample can significantly strengthen the reliability of the findings and applicability in patient and community management.

It is important to consider the fact that there can still be a large reservoir of unidentified characteristics belonging to Sri Lankan *L. donovani* parasites, of which some may be critically important to understand the clinical and epidemiological sequelae, treatment response prediction, and many other aspects that are of importance to disease control.

6.3 IS THE LOCAL INFECTION NEW OR OLD?

It is important to understand whether Sri Lankan parasites were prevalent in the island since long and evolved together with host, vector, and other characteristics or whether they were recently introduced. Following the report of the first few historical cases, leishmaniasis was almost unheard of until 2001, when the onset of the recent outbreak was officially recorded. However, active awareness campaigns and availability of a dermatologist in Southern Sri Lanka resulted in increased case reporting. This increment in case numbers cannot be attributed to the recent emergence of an infection. It is rather possible that an already established *Leishmania* transmission cycle was maintained in Sri Lanka undercover of the unawareness and low transmission. This possibility has been well-thought by the Sri Lankan scientists in the past (Dissanaike, 1981; Wijesundera, 2001). Our more recent research evidence so far also points towards long-term existence of leishmaniasis in Sri Lanka. The case of the British girl as described in the previous chapters supports the assumption that visceralizing strains of *L. donovani* existed in Sri Lanka since long. Historical reports described in previous chapters, the genetically distinct nature of the local parasite, and evidence for established and continued clinico-epidemiological characteristics specific to each transmission focus (Siriwardana, 2008, 2010, 2019, 2020) further favour the long-term existence of the infection within the island.

6.4 WHY LOCAL INFECTION REMAINED UNDETECTED?

Leishmaniasis was not apparent in Sri Lanka until recently. It is interesting and useful to understand why the clinical disease was not detected. Maintenance in the sylvatic cycles which prevented man-vector contact, slow transmission levels in humans, lack of awareness, and suspicion among general public and professional communities may have played a role in this. Anti-malarial insecticide spraying activities which were continued in Sri Lanka aiming at control of malaria transmission would have contributed to maintenance of a low sandfly population within the peri-domestic environments, while limiting leishmaniasis to sylvatic cycles within the island. It is then likely that cessation of these activities along with the reduction of local transmission of malaria and then elimination of the same may have resulted in an increase in insect vector populations, which in turn resulted in increased leishmanial infection among human populations.

The prolonged civil war in Northern Sri Lanka would have brought soldiers in close contact with the sylvatic transmission cycles and eventual infections in them.

6.5 CONCEPT OF CO-EVOLUTION

Many parasites are known to have co-evolved with their hosts. The *L. donovani* complex also has shown a similar behaviour. Members of the genus *Leishmania* have demonstrated geographical variation. Furthermore, there are different hosts and vectors identified in different regions in the world. It is known that isolated populations within a given vertebrate species are likely to get infected with a distinct group of *Leishmania* parasites. Each parasite species within the genus is known to be transmitted by a known single sandfly species. Therefore, existence of *L. donovani* in the island is more likely to be a long-term co-evolution rather than a recent introduction.

In Sri Lanka, *Phlebotomus* spp. sandflies have been identified since long. They are likely to be the potential vector of leishmaniasis in Sri Lanka. However, due to the anthroponotic nature of *L. donovani* and the appearance of large numbers of human infections in closely related communities within a short time, it is very likely that human-to-human transmission is the main mode of transmission of leishmaniasis in Sri Lanka.

6.6 WHERE IS THE ORIGIN OF LOCAL PARASITE?

It is thought that *L. donovani* originated in Africa (Pratlong et al., 2001). Studies on the local parasite provided evidence for their close relationship with Asian parasites (Siriwardana et al., 2007; Kumar et al., 2015). Indian origin was indicated in the historical case of possible PKDL, which would have facilitated an onward propagation of these parasites subsequently in the local setting. Identification of the origin of the Sri Lankan parasite will be of interest. This will have certain implications in understanding the epidemiology of the disease in Sri Lanka.

Sri Lanka had been a popular trade destination to many countries since ancient days. This would have also facilitated acquisition of leishmanial infection from any of these countries. Origin of historical cases since 1904 could be one of these countries. Alternatively, mass migration of people to African countries occurred in 1970s including almost 70,000 individuals in 1983. Majority of them stayed at least for 2 years in these countries (impact of out and return migration on domestic employment of Sri Lanka: the Asian Employment Programme, 1985. Cited in Naotunne et al., 1990).

This mass movement of people may also have contributed to the acquisition of infection from those countries and subsequent establishment of the parasite strains in Sri Lanka, leading to parasite strain propagation at least in a proportion of cases that are seen today.

Though clinical features observed in Northern Sri Lanka (mainly non-ulcerating lesions) are more compatible with the clinical features of *Leishmania tropica* infection as described in subsequent chapters, genotyping of Sri Lankan isolates that mostly included Northern Sri Lankan isolates supported the finding of variant *L. donovani* and partially excludes this possibility.

Irrespective of its unknown origin, the local parasite has shown ominous evidence for its potentially harmful nature. The local cutaneous strains are potentially dangerous as they may visceralize with time. Virulence of parasites may increase during the epidemic (Bucheton et al., 2002) as it has been already clinically observed with the reporting of VL and CL in the country. Lack of gP63 gene expression (Chakrabarty et al., 1996), reduced acid phosphatase activity (Singla et al., 1992), mini-exon genes of chromosome 36 (Zhang et al., 2003), and the parasite strain itself (Dey et al., 2002) are known to affect the level of virulence in *Leishmania*. Genetic basis of unusual phenotypic behaviour of dermotropic *L. donovani* has been further demonstrated with the availability of a complete genome sequence of dermotropic *L. donovani* (Lypaczewski et al., 2018). The recent emergence of visceral leishmaniasis, high level of sero-prevalence in cutaneous leishmaniasis, and poor treatment response patterns already indicate an unpredictable future.

This species confirmation leaves the scientists probably at the doorstep of a new era to begin studying the parasite further and discover all practically and diagnostically important differences, rather than bringing the species research to a conclusion. It is possible that visceralizing *L. donovani* strains of classical visceral leishmaniasis and visceralizing and non-visceralizing *L. donovani* strains of cutaneous leishmaniasis exist in the country.

Epidemiological Aspects 7

Collection of accurate epidemiological information and timely implementation of control activities based on the obtained evidence are important for the success of disease control programmes. Information about where, when, and how people acquire leishmanial infection that may lead to clinical disease can provide important clues to vector behaviour and host-associated transmission dynamics. Leishmaniasis, in particular, sets a typical example of a disease in which the characteristics are diverse, complex, and tend to differ between epidemiological settings. Leishmaniasis disease control programmes when based on local research information and designed on locally suitable disease control strategies are likely to result in better outcomes. Emergence of human leishmaniasis in Sri Lanka led to an urgent need for identification of the transmission dynamics, including distribution, true burden, and risk factors of the disease. This was more so with the continued and increasingly reported case numbers from different locations within the island and the discovery of an unusual parasite variant.

By 2003, it was evident that the majority of cases were from Northern Sri Lanka. The initial studies demonstrated a close association of the disease with outdoor behaviours of the human host (Siriwardana et al., 2003). However, the few historical cases already originated from different and widely geographically diverse areas within the island indicated the possibility of silent and independent transmission cycles in different areas within the island. Furthermore, at least a few cases of leishmaniasis were reported from all three of the main climatic zones ('dry', 'intermediate' and 'wet') from very early stages of the recent epidemic (author's research data base, UCFM). A slow transmission probably occurred in these foci, most probably due to the regular antimalarial vector control activities carried out in the island. The recent outbreak in Northern Sri Lanka would have been the result of the activated passive case detection (APCD) at professional settings in the region following our awareness campaigns.

However, it was not clear as to what disease transmission dynamics exist in the country, whether they were similar throughout the country, if they differ between the various eco-epidemiological settings in the country, or whether

DOI: 10.1201/9781003281801-7

they showed year-on-year variation. Since *Leishmania donovani* is usually transmitted from human to human, at least in the Indian subcontinent, early detection and management of human infection with the parasites can minimize further spread of the infection by reducing the parasite 'reservoirs'. Passive case detection (PCD) is not considered a true reflection of the disease burden. Therefore, it was an urgent necessity to carry out an active case detection programme.

7.1 FIRST FIELD STUDY IN NORTHERN SRI LANKA

Following the first clinical study (2003), Sri Lanka's first active case detection programme was completed in years 2003–2004 in Weli-Oya, a war affected and security-wise a partially uncleared area situated in the country's dry zone in Northern Sri Lanka, during that time (Siriwardana et al., 2010; Siriwardana, 2008). A house-to-house screening campaign was carried out under military cover in this area. The subjects investigated in the study had lived for at least one year in the study area. When surveyed, in 2003, Weli-Oya was still an unsettled area where military activities were common. There were over 20 small or large water reservoirs (*wewa*) in the area, ensuring adequate soil moisture for agriculture. Air temperatures ranged from 26°C to 34°C, and most of the annual rainfall, which varies from 1200 to 1300 mm, falls in the single rainy season. The human communities were interspersed in the scrub jungle, close to thick forest.

In this study, 1386 residents (aged between 1 and 90 years) representing Sampath Nuwara DS division were surveyed, representing 22% of the total population of the study area. Thirty-three patients were detected and a point prevalence of 2.4% (with a 95% confidence interval (CI) of 1.6%–3.2%) was obtained. The prevalence of cutaneous leishmaniasis was higher among the male subjects than among the females (3.7% v. 0.9%), higher among the subjects aged 21–40 years than in the other age-groups, and higher among the security personnel than among the civilians.

In this study, most important risk factors identified by multiple-regression analysis were male gender, spending a mean of ≥5 hours/day in outdoor work, and an age of 20–40 years. In terms of the crude odds ratios, subjects aged 20–40 years had a 3.6-fold higher risk of acquiring cutaneous leishmaniasis than others, and, compared with females, males were more than four times as likely to acquire the disease. Each of these crude odds ratios, obtained in univariate analyses, was only slightly altered when adjustments were made for other factors in multivariate analyses. In the latter analyses, subjects who spent a mean of ≥5 hours, in every 24 hours, in outdoor activities in the area were found to be at a 9.8-fold greater risk of acquiring cutaneous leishmaniasis than those who spent less time for outdoor activities. In this area, an association between age, gender, and occupation was expected because majority of cutaneous leishmaniasis cases identified in Northern Sri Lanka were young male soldiers.

Although the results of the univariate analyses indicated that cutaneous leishmaniasis was particularly common among military personnel and farmers (who, compared with the unemployed subjects, showed 17- and 4-fold higher risk, respectively), neither of these associations reached statistical significance (probably because the sample was small). The total number of people living in a subject's household, ownership of pets and/or farm animals, presence of shelters in the home compound, frequency of visits to animal sheds, and housing conditions (in terms of the nature of walls, the presence of cracks and crevices in walls, and the type of roof) were not found to have any significant effect on the risk of cutaneous leishmaniasis in the study population, further favouring an outdoor transmission.

7.2 FIRST FIELD STUDY IN SOUTHERN SRI LANKA

In the meantime, patients continued to be reported from different geographical locations within the country. Two years later in 2005, a house-to-house screening survey was carried out in Mamadala in the district of Hambantota in the dry zone in Southern Sri Lanka. When investigated, Mamadala was a peaceful, rural domesticated area, where the main occupation was farming. The communities in this area were not located within the scrub jungle. During this survey, 32 cases of cutaneous leishmaniasis were detected among the 938 study participants, giving a point prevalence of 3.4% (CI=2.4%–4.1%). It was interesting to note that at this survey site, there were marked differences in cutaneous leishmaniasis prevalence with age but not with gender or occupation.

The univariate analyses identified three factors; an age between 11 and 40 years, living in a household with five or more members, and the presence of cracks and crevices on the walls of the house. Each factor was associated with a twofold higher risk of acquiring leishmaniasis in the study population. These

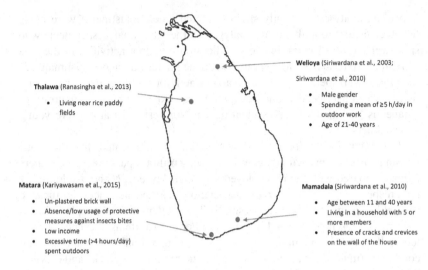

Thalawa (Ranasingha et al., 2013)

- Living near rice paddy fields

Welioya (Siriwardana et al., 2003; Siriwardana et al., 2010)

- Male gender
- Spending a mean of ≥5 h/day in outdoor work
- Age of 21-40 years

Matara (Kariyawasam et al., 2015)

- Un-plastered brick wall
- Absence/low usage of protective measures against insects bites
- Low income
- Excessive time (>4 hours/day) spent outdoors

Mamadala (Siriwardana et al., 2010)

- Age between 11 and 40 years
- Living in a household with 5 or more members
- Presence of cracks and crevices on the wall of the house

FIGURE 7.1 Locations of the field study sites and identified risk factors within the country.

risk levels remained unchanged when multiple logistic regression was applied. None of the other potential risk factors investigated (i.e., gender, occupation, time spent outdoors, and the presence of animals or animal shelters) was found to be significantly associated with a risk for cutaneous leishmaniasis, indicating a peri-domestic nature of disease transmission.

A third and a small-scale study was carried out during the same period in Kataragama, a village situated in the district of Moneragala in Southern Sri Lanka (Siriwardana et al., 2010), (Figure 7.1).

The climatic conditions and geography of Kataragama are similar to those of Mamadala. Although Weli-oya and Mamadala were known case-prevalent areas (author's patient data base), no cases of leishmaniasis had been reported in Kataragama prior to this study. Interestingly, one case of cutaneous leishmaniasis was identified, confirmed by light microscopy of lesion scrapings, giving a prevalence of 0.5% in this area.

In the meantime, case referrals to our weekly leishmaniasis clinic continued and represented almost all the provinces by 2008 (author's patient database). There were slight differences of the figures relating to our activated passive case detection data due to the case referral patterns and levels of initial case suspicion at the first health care contact level. Except for that, case distribution maps based on our referral data indicated a gradual expansion of spatial distribution. However, most numbers of patients were identified from Northern and Southern provinces every year. Analysis of these cases revealed a seasonal distribution of case presentation with two peaks in early and late months of the year that was apparent (Siriwardana et al., 2019). Analysis of annual data indicated that this bi-annual pattern existed from the beginning and at each focus in the North and the South in an independent manner (Siriwardana et al., 2010). The higher cutaneous leishmaniasis incidence pattern seen in early months and later months of every year correlates well with the monsoonal rainy seasons in the island.

Leishmaniasis was declared a notifiable disease in Sri Lanka by the Ministry of Health, in 2008.

However, case reporting data based on passive case detections (PCDs) or activated passive case detections (APCDs) do not always reflect the true situation, though they are often used as projections of the actual situation. Multiple factors including the rate of disease transmission, host factors, level of self-referral, awareness, and capacity in case detection can greatly influence the variation between the actually existing number of infected cases in the community and those detected at health care settings. Therefore, large-scale active case detection (ACD) programmes were of timely importance.

In the subsequent years, two more studies have been carried out in Northern and Southern Sri Lanka.

7.3 SUBSEQUENT FIELD STUDIES

The fourth study covering a case-prevalent area in Northern Sri Lanka was reported by one of our fellow institutions in 2013, 10 years after the first study in Northern Sri Lanka (Ranasinghe et al., 2013). A cross-sectional study had been carried out, covering 954 participants of an estimated population of 61,674 to identify cases of cutaneous leishmaniasis and asymptomatic visceral leishmaniasis, and risk factors for transmission. A total of 31 cases of cutaneous leishmaniasis and one healthy individual with positive rK39 rapid diagnostic test result were detected during this attempt. Living near paddy fields ($P \leq 0.01$) was a risk factor identified in this study for transmission of cutaneous leishmaniasis. This probably indicated an outdoor nature of disease transmission.

Our recent study covering the whole district of Matara was conducted during 2013–2014 to obtain scientific evidence representative of a larger geographical area in Sri Lanka (Kariyawasam et al., 2015). This study reported evidence for peri-domestic transmission in the study area. A total of 2260 individuals from four divisional secretariat divisions (DSDs, an administrative sub division within a district) were screened by house-to-house surveys, and 38 cases of cutaneous leishmaniasis were detected, giving a disease prevalence of 1.68%. The study population had an age range of 1–90 years (median=43±17.31), a low monthly income (<20,000 LKR, 52.8%), and a male-to-female ratio of 1:2.

Significant case clustering with proximity to forest areas was observed in this study. Un-plastered brick walls, absence or low usage of protective measures against insect bites, low income, and excessive time (>4 hours/day) spent outdoors were identified as risk factors. These findings can be considered as early evidence for peri-domestication of a sylvatic transmission cycle.

7.4 POSSIBILITY OF LOCAL ANIMAL RESERVOIRS

Meanwhile, preliminary evidence for possible animal reservoir hosts has also been highlighted in Sri Lanka. A study from central Sri Lanka examined 151 samples of canine serum collected from patient areas in 15 villages in Central, North Western, and North Central provinces in Sri Lanka (Nawaratna et al., 2009). Two samples have demonstrated *Leishmania* amastigotes in Giemsa-stained smears of the skin and of peripheral blood, respectively. Rodents [one Ceylon gerbril (*Tatera indica indica*), 12 bandicoots (*Bandicota indicaindica*), and 34 black rats (*Rattus rattus*)] did not show evidence for *Leishmania* infection. In the second study, sera from 114 dogs have been examined by the canine immunochromatographic strip assays based on recombinant K39 antigen. Anti-*Leishmania spp.* antibodies were detectable in 1/114 (0.9%) dogs (Rosypal et al., 2010). Isolation of *Leishmania* parasites in slit scrapings of skin and peripheral blood from two dogs and detection of rK39 sero-positivity in one dog in two different occasions provide preliminary evidence for animal involvement in leishmaniasis transmission.

7.5 SINGLE OR MULTIPLE MODES OF PARASITE MAINTENANCE AND TRANSMISSION?

Five active case detection programmes have been conducted up to date in the island so far, at different geo-locations. These included different time intervals and covered four districts in Northern and Southern Sri Lanka,

Anuradhapura, Hambantota, Moneragala, and Matara (Figure 7.1). Weli-oya study was the first detailed survey conducted to measure the prevalence of cutaneous leishmaniasis and investigated the associated risk factors in selected areas within Northern Sri Lanka. The relatively high prevalence recorded in the area soon after the detection of the epidemic indicated already-established disease transmission in the area. Observations made during early years in other two areas in Southern Sri Lanka are also indicative of well-established local transmission in these areas, both of which had previously been identified as foci of human leishmaniasis in our historical reports (Castellani et al., 1904; Chapman, 1973; Dissanaike, 1981; Athukorale et al., 1992; Siriwardana et al., 2007).

In the first study area, more males than females were engaged in outdoor activities, such as military activities and farming, especially in the hours between dusk and dawn, when most transmission probably occurs (Al-Tawfiq et al., 2004). The predominance of male cases and the absence of cases aged <20 years possibly reflected the minimal indoor or peri-domestic transmission. Association of the disease with young adulthood, male gender, and time spent outdoors would have been probably due to the nature of human behaviours that increased the exposure of themselves to the sandfly vectors.

It seems possible that the causative parasite was maintained in a sylvatic/ zoonotic cycle in this area. This view, however, contradicts the popular belief that the transmission of *L. donovani* is largely anthroponotic in Asia. Preliminary evidence found with regard to animal reservoirs supported an existing zoonotic cycle. In contrast, Ranasinghe et al. did not identify any significant association with animals in the study area in Northern Sri Lanka. The authors have suggested the possibility of the presence of non-canine reservoirs. They further highlighted small mammal species (i.e., *Rattus* spp.), which were identified as reservoir hosts for other *Leishmania spp.* (i.e., *Leishmania major*) and *Canis aureus*, an identified reservoir host of *L. infantum*, that are present in Sri Lanka, could be potential reservoir hosts (Arudpragasam et al., 1982). Authors in their report further suggest a peri-domestic transmission cycle for leishmaniasis in the Northern study area. Subsequent peri-domestication of an initially zoonotic transmission cycle could be a possibility. Supporting this, sandfly vectors *(described in forthcoming chapters)* have been identified in a range of peri-domestic breeding and resting sites (decaying garbage, unclear areas, termite hills, and wet soil) with increased odds for disease transmission (Wijerathna et al., 2020).

The incidence and/or spread of leishmaniasis can be escalated by civil unrest and war activities (Reyburn et al., 2003). A long civil war was ongoing for several years in Northern Sri Lanka may have played a role in this. Poor socioeconomic and nutritional conditions, large numbers of military personnel working outdoors, deforestation, and the restructuring of certain areas for security reasons may have all contributed to the increasing incidence and possible peri-domestication of cutaneous leishmaniasis in the North.

In contrast to the findings obtained in Northern Sri Lankan studies, people residing in survey sites in Southern Sri Lanka appeared to be at the highest risk of acquiring leishmanial infection when in peri-domestic environments. Case clustering was also evident in the more recent large-scale study (Kariyawasam et al., 2015). In anthroponotic foci of leishmaniasis, household and other small-scale, spatial clustering of cases is often observed (Bern et al., 2000; Desjeux, 2001; Bucheton et al., 2002; Ranjan et al., 2005; Schenkel et al., 2006). Human-to-human transmission can be enhanced by the presence of a peri-domestic vector. Studies in the South were carried out several years later, following the Northern Sri Lankan study. It is possible that a sylvatic and a zoonotic cycle (as apparent in North) initially existed in South also and expanded through spread of the parasites and vectors to a peri-domestic environment, resulting in an anthroponotic cycle (Desjeux, 2001; Baldi et al., 2004).

Field detection of a case of cutaneous leishmaniasis in an area with no reported cases during our field study in South highlighted the importance of active screening. The early detection and treatment of cases in areas with low disease prevalence helps prevent significant outbreaks.

The possibility of regional variation in the mode of transmission of the parasites causing cutaneous leishmaniasis within Sri Lanka is supported by previous observations on the varying behaviour of *Phlebotomus argentipes*, the local vector (Lewis et al., 1973; Lane et al., 1990) as well as by the recently carried out clinical studies (Siriwardana et al., 2010, 2019). Both morphospecies A and B of *P. argentipes* have been detected in Northern Sri Lanka (Surendran et al., 2005), but only morphospecies B appears to be associated with the anthroponotic transmission of *L. donovani* in endemic areas of India.

7.6 SHORT AND LONG TERM IMPLICATIONS

Presence of human leishmaniasis in Sri Lanka can have many socioeconomic implications. The large-scale, post-war redevelopment activities now taking place and the increasing number of cases of cutaneous leishmaniasis, often clustered in space and time, can significantly favour the onward transmission of the parasites, particularly the anthroponotic transmission. Free movement of non-immune people to existing foci may also help maintain the disease (Reyburn et al., 2003). With a major thrust towards the promotion of tourism in the post-war era, leishmaniasis in Sri Lanka has already posed a threat to non-immune travellers from other countries (Ito et al., 2014).

Regional variation in transmission characteristics within the country will probably complicate preventive activities. Scientific information, especially on the vector and possible reservoir hosts, is urgently required.

Potential for the local vector to develop insecticide resistance has also been identified recently (Surendran et al., 2005). Irrational use of insecticides has been shown to result in undesired sequelae, including insecticide resistance in the past (Sanyal et al., 1979). The beneficial effects of sandfly control in the numerous Old-World foci of zoonotic cutaneous leishmaniasis have often been transient. Timely treatment of humans and dogs in such foci is recommended (Desjeux, 1992). Studies to identify sand fly gut microbiota for paratransgenesis, a vector-based method of control of *Leishmania* parasites, have shown encouraging results (Gunathilaka et al., 2020).

Once the full characteristics of the Sri Lankan leishmaniasis are known, an integrated control programme may be designed. Integrated control is a concept that is currently receiving much attention in the Indian subcontinent (Dujardin, 2006; Chappuis et al., 2007; Ostyn et al., 2008; Mondal et al., 2009). Programmes of active case detection will minimize underreporting (Bern et al., 2008). In the meantime, the focus should be on adopting general preventive measures, strengthening case management, and further research in all relevant areas.

Vectors and Reservoir Hosts

8

Role of sandflies as vectors in leishmaniasis was first confirmed in 1942 in India (Swaminath et al., 2006). Female sandfly vectors belonging to two genera, *Phlebotomus* in the old world and *Lutzomyia* in the new world, are responsible for transmission of leishmaniasis in a range of hosts through infective bites. Out of the many hundreds of Phlebotomine species described so far, only about 30 are incriminated in the transmission of leishmaniasis in the old world (Bates, 2007). The female sandflies are blood suckers from human or many vertebrate animals. Blood meal is necessary for ovulation and egg development in the sandflies. They get infected with *Leishmania spp.* during a blood meal from an infected host. Following ingestion by the vector, amastigote stages of the parasite transform into promastigote stage over a period of several days, and multiplication follows in the gut. Subsequent blood meal introduces the infective stages of parasites to the new host and transmission cycle is completed (Bates, 2007).

8.1 GEOGRAPHY-BASED COMPLEXITIES

Spatial distribution of both the disease and its sandfly vectors in different parts of the world are known to be widening as a result of continued attempts of the parasite and the vector to adopt to the changing environment (Sukra et al., 2013; Srinivasan et al., 2014; Sharma et al., 2005; Uranw et al., 2013; Gonzalez et al., 2010). Therefore, it is important to identify the vector species, their spatial and temporal distribution, and the level of contribution to leishmaniasis transmission in an endemic setting. Identification of their behaviours, insecticide susceptibility, and other characteristics is also important in each endemic

DOI: 10.1201/9781003281801-8

setting in order to determine the disease transmission dynamics and design disease control strategies.

Phlebotomus argentipes, (Annandale Brunetti) is a widely distributed insect in the Indian subcontinent, Southeast Asian region, and many parts of the world (Lane et al., 1986, 1990). It is known as the incriminated vector of *Leishmania donovani* in India. Phlebotomine vectors were known to have a wider geographical distribution, extending from Iran and Afghanistan in West and extending to Malaysia and Indonesia in the SEA region since long (Lewis et al., 1973). In spite of this, occurrence or at least the reported distribution of visceral leishmaniasis was restricted to some parts of India (Ilango et al., 1994). Sri Lanka too did not have or at least did not report leishmaniasis until the recent past. It was thought that variable susceptibility levels of different vector populations to *L. donovani* is the probable reason for this difference.

8.2 SANDFLY VECTORS IN SRI LANKA

Phlebotomus argentipes sandfly vectors of leishmaniasis have been described in Sri Lanka since long (Brunetti, 1912; Carter et al., 1949; Lewis, 1978; Lane et al., 1990). Morphological differences in at least five subgroups within the species found in Sri Lanka had also been demonstrated since long (Lewis, 1978; Lane, 1980). Sandfly abundance in different geographical settings was also known (Lewis et al., 1973; Surendran et al., 2005a, 2005b). Female counterparts of sandflies were reported to be zoophilic in many areas (Lewis et al., 1973) but appeared mainly anthropophagic elsewhere (Lane et al., 1990).

Rarity of the disease in Sri Lanka in spite of its vector abundance was initially attributed to the zoophilic nature of the then identified sandfly vectors in the island (Lewis et al., 1973). Different behaviour patterns of the sandfly including this factor and differences in the degree of anthropophagy were also suggested as possible reasons (Lewis et al., 1973). However, in 1988, Lane concluded that sandflies prevalent in Central highlands were probably anthropophilic (Lane et al., 1990). This study further revealed that biting rates in study areas were similar to those reported in India, where visceral leishmaniasis was already considered endemic during that time. These findings supported the low transmission levels existing in Sri Lanka as the reason for rarity of the disease. Rarity was probably due to antimalarial measures or the sylvatic nature of the disease or both. More recent studies have identified a range of non-sylvatic sandfly breeding and resting sites interspersed in human settlements and their associations with increased odds of leishmaniasis transmission (Wijerathna et al., 2020).

Many morphological and genetic-based studies on sandfly taxonomy have been carried out in Sri Lanka. With the recent emergence (or recent discovery) of cutaneous leishmaniasis in the country, local scientists have undertaken further studies on sandfly vectors. First, such a report on attempts toward morphological characterization of *Phlebotomus argentipes* was published in 2005 (Surendran et al., 2005). Authors were able to collect the flies using human traps and further proved the anthropophagic nature of the sandflies in Northern Sri Lanka and in Southern Sri Lanka (in Delft islands and Moneragala, respectively).

They reported the presence of two morphospecies A and B of *Phlebotomus argentipes sensu lato* in Sri Lanka based on the morphological differences. Some morphological differences were known to correlate with the extent of visceral leishmaniasis occurrence in India and used to differentiate between sandfly species (e.g., length of *Sensilla chaetica*) (Lane et al., 1986). Morphospecies identified in this study are already known to possess different vectoral capacities. Morphospecies B, which is associated with visceral leishmaniasis in India, was identified in Northern Sri Lanka, while the flies collected from South belonged to morphospecies A, which is not known to be associated with visceral leishmaniasis transmission. Only morphospecies A had been reported in Sri Lanka previously (Lewis et al., 1973; Lane et al., 1990).

Subsequently, sandflies collected from the Delft island in Northern Sri Lanka were genetically identified to be *Phlebotomus argentipes* Annandale & Brunetti, the primary vector in India and anthropophagic and zoophagic populations were also identified. With this finding, authors speculated this species to be the most likely vector in Sri Lanka.

During this period, the main clinical form of leishmaniasis continued to be cutaneous leishmaniasis in spite of our finding of *L. donovani* which is transmitted anthroponotically (Siriwardana et al., 2008). Anthroponotic cutaneous leishmaniasis (AnCL) is mainly caused by *Leishmania tropica* and transmitted by *Phlebotomus sergenti* and *Phlebotomus papatasi* (Kalra et al., 1986), while the findings in Sri Lanka were different. Further insight into this can be obtained from the findings of subsequent studies conducted by same local researchers (Surendran et al., 2007). Attempts have been made to describe sandfly prevalence and socio-environmental factors leading to man–vector transmission of *Leishmania* in Northern Sri Lanka in this study (Surendran et al., 2007). The study was conducted in the Delft island in Northern Sri Lanka. There was no awareness on leishmaniasis or the potential role of sandflies as vectors in transmitting the disease. Authors highlighted the need for raising awareness. The same study identified sandfly larvae from cracks of mud floors of house favouring an indoor transmission. They further described the presence of environmental conditions that are conducive to vector prevalence, including crevices in the uniquely constructed parapet-walls made of local coral-stones, highly humid and dry grey loam soil, and extensive growth of pasture grass in the study areas.

Prevalence of *P. argentipes* in the dry zone, wet zone, and coastal belts in the dry zone in Sri Lanka during years 2005–2006 had been reported by other scientists as well (Ozbel et al., 2011). Presence of *P. santoni* and *Sergentomyia* species were also reported in this study.

Few years later, taxonomy of *P. argentipes* complex in the Asian region was re-assessed and presence of three species, viz., *Phlebotomus glaucus*, *P. argentipes sensu stricto*, and *P. annandalei* was confirmed by morphological means (Ilango, 2010). Complexity of a species and presence of multiple taxa in an endemic setting can alter and conceal the actual disease transmission patterns, leading to incorrect observations and therefore inaccuracy in decisions on vector control activities. The accurate and reliable definition of vectors and their bionomics are important for a successful vector control programme especially when the vector taxon exists as a species complex. Filling further gaps in local knowledge, morphospecies identification data in Sri Lanka (Surendran et al., 2005) have also been re-examined few years later (Gajapathy et al., 2011). A study carried out in Jaffna mainland and two associated islands in Northern Sri Lanka has reported all three members of the complex. *P. glaucus* and *P. argentipes s.s.* were reported for the first time in Sri Lanka in this study. Considering the difficulties associated with morphological characterization of vectors, the authors further suggested employment of molecular means for the characterization of the sandfly vectors.

Soon after, a fourth distinct population of sandflies from Matale in Central Sri Lanka was identified by morphological means (Ranasinghe et al., 2012). This new population was different form all three previously identified members of the complex; *P. argentipes sensu lato*, *P. glaucus*, and *P. annandelei*. Further attempts on identification of this member have not been recorded in literature so far. Findings so far indicated the complexity of the sandfly vector species complex that exist within the country. It will be useful to conduct a genetic assessment using appropriate genetic tools on a sandfly population that adequately represent all the regions in the island, study of their behaviours, and the role as vectors of *Leishmania*.

Gajapathy et al. (2013), making further attempts to achieve a better taxonomic understanding, carried out a study covering sandfly populations in different parts of Sri Lanka, including patient localities, to characterize the sibling species of *Phlebotomus* (*Euphlebotomus*) *argentipes sensu lato* and to establish their possible role in *Leishmania* transmission using molecular means. Vector sampling has covered multiple areas from the dry zone both in Northern and Southern Sri Lanka.

Multiple genetic targets have been examined in this study (cytochrome oxidase subunit I (CO I), cytochrome oxidase b (cyt b), and internal transcribed spacer 2 (ITS2) and 18s and 28s rDNA). Analysis of genetic targets confirmed the species as *P. argentipes* complex. However, the three groups proposed by morphological means previously were found in only two genetically distinct groups, (A and B). Furthermore, authors identified *Leishmania* DNA [mini-circle kinetoplastid, heat shock protein 70 (hsp70) and internal transcribed spacer I DNA] and human blood from sibling species A which had not been known to transmit leishmaniasis until that time. *P. argentipes* morpho species A was introduced as a potential vector of leishmaniasis in Sri Lanka in this study.

Incrimination of a new sibling species of vector carries great importance. Behaviours of these variants may also be different from that of known members. It is necessary to understand these behaviours and define exact roles of each sibling species in disease transmission.

Further studies conducted in Sri Lanka (Senanayake et al., 2015) has further confirmed the finding of *P.. argentipes glaucus* (*P.. argentipes* morpho species A) in some parts of the country. Blood meal analysis confirmed the presence of *L. donovani* DNA. A non-vector species, *Sergentomyia zeylanica,* was also identified in this study. *S. zeylanica* was considered a biting nuisance, has an anthropophilic nature, and was not known to transmit leishmaniasis. The peak aggregation period of sandflies was identified as 8:00 PM to 11:00 PM (Senanayake et al., 2015).

Further attempts on accurate identification of the locally prevalent sandflies using molecular biological tools revealed interesting findings (Gajapathy et al., 2016). Taxonomical studies based on cytochrome c oxidase gene subunit 1 (COI) sequence and subsequent barcoding on 70 samples collected from dry zone areas in Northern and Southern Sri Lanka (districts of Hambantota, Anuradhapura, Vavuniya, Trincomalee and Jaffna) have shown existence of multiple species. The study further confirmed the accuracy of morphology-based identification. Furthermore, the analysis delineated morphologically identified *Sergentomyia bailyi, S babu babu,* and *S babu insularis* into genetically distinct groups.

During this time, a study conducted in India revealed the presence of species complex within the *S. bailyi* (Yogeswari et al., 2016). Sri Lankan researchers further attempted examining the same possibility in the local setting. These attempts revealed for the first time morphological and genetic evidence for the presence of two cryptic species within the *S. bailyi* complex in Sri Lanka as well (Tharmatha et al., 2017).

8.3 INSECTICIDE RESISTANCE

Along with the complexity of the local sandfly populations identified in the taxonomic studies, it is important to note the preliminary evidence provided for insecticide resistance during the early period of the epidemic. Surendran et al. (2005) assayed the sandflies for activities of four enzyme systems involved in insecticide resistance (acetylcholinesterase, nonspecific carboxylesterases, glutathione-S-transferases, and cytochrome p450 monooxygenases). The work revealed preliminary evidence for elevated esterases and altered acetylcholinesterase, indicating possibility of insecticide resistance. This was thought to be due to long-lasting antimalarial activities in the region using spraying of malathion-based insecticides. Insecticide resistance in *P. argentipes* Annandale and Brunetti, the vector of kala-azar in the Indian subcontinent, was first reported in 1987 in Bihar in India. Irrational use of insecticides has brought about devastating results in the past (Sanyal et al., 1979).

8.4 INFORMATION ADEQUACY AND GAPS AND NEEDS

It is noteworthy to mention that Sri Lanka already possesses a significant amount of information on vectors, especially on the vector incrimination aspects. Complexity of the sandfly population, potential for insecticide resistance, and wide prevalence of vectors are important concerns. Comprehensive studies on identification of the sandfly behaviours, possible regional variations as already shown with regard to other characteristics within the focus (Siriwardana et al., 2010, 2019; Kariyawasam et al., 2015), and insecticide susceptibility parameters will be of timely importance. Though it is generally believed that *P. argentipes* is found in peri-domestic environments and the control activities have been based on these assumptions failed too, exophillic *P. argentipes* have been reported to have high human biting rates at the same time (Poche et al., 2011). Strengthening laboratory and field entomological capacity will be of importance.

The spatial distribution of both the disease and its vectors is widening as a result of their continued attempts to adopt to the changing scenarios of the environment at a global scale. Insecticide-based control of sandflies is a major component in vector control activities used in many countries. However, emergence of insecticide resistance is one such adaptation demonstrated by sandflies in many countries (Karakus et al., 2017; Shirani-Bidabadi et al., 2017; Cetin et al., 2017).

Many reports originating from Asia indicate that antimalarial spraying has benefited leishmaniasis control activities. In India, national antimalarial activities that included DDT spraying is thought to result in a reduction of reported patient numbers or sandfly populations (Kaul et al., 1994; Pandya, 1983; Nadim et al., 1970). Emergence of insecticide resistance in sandflies can result in a serious impact on disease control. Continued surveillance of the outcome of natural and human activities is necessary in such a situation.

It has been suggested to use different classes of insecticides in rotation (e.g., pyrethroids instead of DDT), mosaics, or a mixture of unrelated ones to prevent or delay emerging insecticide resistance (Dhiman et al., 2016). Integrated control activities where vector control is combined with other means is a promising option considered in many endemic countries now.

There is a need for properly obtained scientific information that will pave the way for decision-making in vector control activities in Sri Lanka. There is a lack of adequate information on the susceptibility of sandflies to insecticides used locally. Also, the vector prevalence and behaviour need to be studied in more depth. Their exact role in disease transmission except for blood meal analyses will be of importance. Once such activities are planned and designed, proper launching together with adequate surveillance methods and preparedness for alternative tools which could be in operation from the onset are of importance. Changes in vector populations both by genetic and behavioural means and also surveillance for emergence of insecticide resistance or adaptation for the changing ecology, environment, or the man-made changes, including control activities, will enable timely revisions in the activities.

Immunological Aspects

9

Identification of a genetically variant *Leishmania donovani* as the cause of cutaneous leishmaniasis in Sri Lanka indicated the possibility of having immuno-pathogenic mechanisms that are different from those associated with traditional cutaneous or visceral leishmaniasis causing species. These differences are very likely to result in differences in lesional and systemic response patterns of host against *L. donovani* infection. Previous reports on atypical lesions, presence of rapid and slow progressing different patterns in classical lesions, poorly responding infections to standard antimony treatment, and emergence of visceral leishmaniasis further indicated this possibility and left the scientists with many questions. Some of them still remain unanswered (at the time of preparation of this chapter). Few studies addressing either *in situ* or systemic responses and underlying causative mechanisms are available in local literature.

Balance between the immuno-pathological reactions raised by the host and the response of the infecting parasite towards these reactions determine the final outcome of an infection. Different components in both innate and adaptive immune systems play different roles in the battle against the establishment of *Leishmania* in the host. This has been widely studied in different clinical forms and parasite forms of leishmaniasis at a global scale. The complement system plays an important role in *Leishmania* elimination by lysing the cells and neutrophils (Moreno et al., 2007) by directly engulfing the parasites (Mollinedo et al., 2010) or by activating an array of chemokines (Charmoy et al., 2007) or natural killer cells (Muller et al., 2001) by producing interferon (IFN) (Scharton et al., 1993) and restricting dissemination (Laskay et al., 1995). *L. donovani* promastigotes (Hoover et al., 1984) and metacyclic promastigotes (Puentes et al., 1988) are known to be more resistant to complement-mediated lysis. NK cells are important in containment of *L. donovani* parasites (Satoskar et al., 1999). There are no Sri Lankan studies addressing the role of innate immunity in response to dermotropic *L. donovani* so far.

First-line cellular resistance exerted by the host in response to *Leishmania* infection is often due to the cellular immune response resulting in macrophage

DOI: 10.1201/9781003281801-9

activation and a leishmanicidal effect (Bousoffara et al., 2004). Cells of adaptive immunity are mainly lymphocytes. It is known that cutaneous leishmaniasis usually results in a cell-mediated response which often confines the establishment of infection and clinical features to the skin, while visceral infection results in a humoral response. Cellular response against intra-cellular pathogens is mainly a Th1 cytokine response.

In extracellular pathogens, a humoral immunity mediated by elevated Th2 cytokine response has been observed (Ulett et al., 2000). Interferon (IFN)-γ produced by CD4+T cells controls parasite multiplication during the early infection in leishmaniasis (Antonelli et al., 2005; Bottrel et al., 2001), whereas CD8+T cells contribute to IFN-γ production and the differentiation of Th1 responses. Predominant Th1 response that results in elevated IFN-γ and IL-2 levels is associated with resistance to leishmaniasis, while a Th2 response resulting in high IL-4 and IL-10 levels indicates susceptibility (Rodrigues et al., 2016; Rodriguez et al., 2007).

Visceralization and dissemination in cutaneous leishmaniasis (diffuse cutaneous leishmaniasis, DCL) have been shown to be associated with insufficient Th1 cytokine response to control infection (Saporito et al., 2013). Cure of visceral leishmaniasis is also shown to be associated with a sustained Th1 response (Portela et al., 2018).

On the other hand, IL-10 is considered the major mediator of the immunological defects observed in the spleen during chronic visceral leishmaniasis (Kumar et al., 2012). IL-10 acts as a major mediator of immunological defects seen in VL. It has been shown that reduction of IL-10 levels or blockade of IL-10 signalling results in increased resistance to *L. donovani* infection (Murphy et al., 2001; Murray et al., 2003).

9.1 *IN SITU* LESIONAL RESPONSE PATTERNS

Research on immunological aspects in Sri Lanka is fairly recent. There are only a few studies addressing the *in situ* host response, humoral response, and host genetics in local *L. donovani* infection.

First study describing cellular immune pathology identified leishmaniasis as a spectral disease similar to leprosy (Herath et al., 2010). Histological findings in a range of cutaneous leishmaniasis infections were identified to be similar to those of the spectrum in leprosy ranging from lepromatous to tuberculoid leprosy. Histological groups showed a significant inverse relationship with the mean parasitic index. The mean percentage T cells showed a variation similar to that seen in leprosy, while mean percentage B cells showed less variation.

A limited number of parasite isolates from cutaneous leishmaniasis and visceral leishmaniasis infections acquired in Sri Lanka were investigated in 2013 (McCall et al., 2013). They demonstrated cutaneous leishmaniasis–induced immunological protection against subsequent visceral infection in the mouse model. Protection was associated with a mixed Th1/Th2 response. Authors further suggested that this cross-immunity as a protective factor resulting in the rarity of visceral leishmaniasis in Sri Lanka.

Variable immune response patterns that are dependent on the treatment response and duration of the lesions have been demonstrated (Manamperi et al., 2017). Localized skin lesions showed significant upregulation of the Th1 cytokine IFN-γ and downregulation of the Th2 cytokine IL-4 in this study. Chronic lesions (duration > 6 months) showed an elevated tissue expression of IFN-γ and TNF-α. Expression of IL-4 was higher in lesions that had poor response to standard antimony therapy. Healing lesions mainly demonstrated a prominent Th1 response, while poorly responding cases had a Th2-associated response.

Presence of antigenic differences between dermotropic and visceralizing *L. donovani* is a possibility that requires careful consideration. Usefulness of a new rapid diagnostic immune-chromatographic strip (CL-Detect™ IC-RDT) has been examined recently (De Silva et al., 2017). The assay that traditionally captures the peroxidoxin antigen of *Leishmania* amastigotes showed very low sensitivity (36%) as compared to PCR detection. Authors concluded that IC-RDT is not suitable to diagnose cutaneous leishmaniasis in Sri Lanka. Even though this study was aimed at examination of the usefulness of this tool in diagnosis, the findings seem to have provided indirect evidence for differential antigen production or expression in local *Leishmania* parasites at the cellular level.

Kariyawasam et al. (2017) demonstrated cytokine (IL-10; IFN-γ) release patterns of mice splenocytes and lymph node cell cultures. Significantly high IFN-γ response associated with cutaneous leishmaniasis, and increased IL-10 levels in visceral leishmaniasis were observed in this study.

Kahandawaarachchi et al. (2017) reported an elevated level of inflammatory markers in a patient with a *Leishmania* parasite positive skin ulcer. He was confirmed to have co-infected with melioidosis. Therefore, the cause for this immunological finding remains uncertain.

9.2 HUMORAL RESPONSE PATTERNS

Significantly elevated and disease-specific humoral response patterns in leish-maniasis are mainly described for visceral leishmaniasis (Lima et al., 2017; Magalhaes et al., 2017; Rodrigues, et al., 2016), while sero-prevalence described in traditionally cutaneous leishmaniasis causing species is usually variable and often low (Pedral-Sampaio et al., 2017; Zeyrek et al., 2007; Sarkari et al., 2014; Szargiki et al., 2009; Hartzell et al., 2008). Similar response patterns have been described in cutaneous leishmaniasis caused by *L. donovani* (Svobodova et al., 2009; Sharma et al., 2009). Furthermore, antigenic differences are also known to exist between members of the same species that are prevalent in different geographical locations (Bhattacharyya et al., 2014, 2013).

During the early stages of the epidemic in Sri Lanka, patients with cutaneous leishmaniasis were screened using formol gel test (FGT) to rule out these possibilities (Siriwardena et al., 2003; Siriwardana, 2008). FGT is a simple screening test that detects markedly increased serum protein levels which can be seen in many systemic infections, including visceral leishmaniasis. Other more specific and more sensitive tools were not available to us during that time. However, these preliminary investigations revealed that there was no evidence of increased serum protein levels. This finding coupled with the absence of systemic manifestations during that time urged us to strongly believe that locally found *L. donovani* are dermotropic and are only capable of producing skin infections.

However, the first case of locally acquired visceral leishmaniasis that was identified in 2005 (published only later with long-term follow-up data in Siriwardana et al., 2017) prompted us to predict the possibility of visceraliza-tion at least in a proportion of cases. Therefore, later on with the availability of better infrastructure, more specific diagnostic tools were employed in screening for a humoral response. Analysis of cases of cutaneous leishmaniasis with rK39 assay revealed no evidence of positivity in the study group, further strengthening the localized nature of cutaneous leishmaniasis (Siriwardana et al., 2010). However, due to the genetically distinct nature of the local *L. donovani* variants, still unidentified antigenic differences at the genetics level leading to differential production or at the expression level leading to strong or weak assay positivity were possibilities. These were addressed by examination of local skin infection with locally developed tools.

An in-house ELISA based on the local crude antigen of dermotropic *Leishmania* spp. showing an 80% sero-prevalence and 100% sero-prevalence observed in visceral leishmaniasis when examined with locally developed assays indicate an early systemic involvement as one possibility. However, findings of Siriwardana et al. (2007), Alam et al. (2009), Kariyawasam et al. (2017), and

Zhang et al. (2014) indicate the presence of a distinct visceralizing parasitic variant. The patients we studied did not show clinical evidence of visceralization. Current sero- prevalence, therefore, most likely favours the former possibility.

Further supporting this, only two of seven (2/7) reported cases of recently identified (or at least formally reported) visceral leishmaniasis (Siriwardana et al., 2017) demonstrated rK39 positivity. This draws the attention to the possibility of antigenic differences between local and known *L. donovani*.

9.3 CASE FOR PARASITOLOGICAL REASONS

More recently, however, parasitological reasons for dermotropism have come into light. Natural attenuation of the parasite and the lack of visceralization of dermotropic cutaneous leishmaniasis variants in humans and in murine models were demonstrated recently. Long-term follow-up of large numbers of adequately treated cases of cutaneous leishmaniasis have not shown clinical features suggestive of visceralization. The study included a 4-year follow-up of 250 cases of laboratory-confirmed cutaneous leishmaniasis (Kariyawasam et al., 2017). Intra- dermal injection of BALB/c mice with cutaneous leishmaniasis strains resulted in the development of cutaneous lesions at the site of inoculation with no signs of systemic dissemination, while intra-dermal injection of traditionally visceralizing *L. donovani* reference strain caused infection in internal organs. Cytokine (IL-10, IFN-γ) release patterns of mice splenocytes and lymph node cell cultures revealed significantly high IFN-γ response associated with cutaneous leishmaniasis and increased IL-10 levels in visceral leishmaniasis. *In vitro* macrophage experiments showed a reduction in the capability to cause infection, rate of growth, and reduced survival of local cutaneous leishmaniasis strains in comparison to reference visceral *Leishmania* strains. Zhang et al. (2014) in their studies further provided supportive evidence for parasitological reasons for the dermotropism.

9.4 ROLE OF HOST GENETICS

Host genetic factors have also been considered on many occasions as an important determinant of the disease pathology and therefore the clinical outcome in leishmaniasis in other parts of the world (Ribas-Silva et al., 2015;

Sakthianandeswaren et al., 2009; Mishra et al., 2015; Blackwell et al., 2009; Ejghal et al., 2014).

Human leukocyte antigen (HLA) genes of class I and II located within the MHC are known to play a role in presenting antigens to CD8+and CD4+T cells. However, studies on HLA genes in Asian populations are scarce and had mainly addressed the associations with visceral leishmaniasis (Amit et al., 2017), while most cutaneous leishmaniasis studies have been carried out in the new world (Castellucci et al., 2014; Lara et al., 1991; Cabrera et al., 1995; Ribaz-Silva et al., 2015). Healing cutaneous lesions in leishmaniasis are known to demonstrate high MHC class 1 restricted CD4+T cells (Silveira et al., 2004).

Samaranayake et al. (2008) reported the presence of significantly high numbers of multiple lesions in cutaneous leishmaniasis among family members in Sri Lanka (P=0.002). However, the study has failed to demonstrate any associated systemic manifestation or a strong overall family association.

A subsequent study which was reported 2 years later investigated the association between selected single-nucleotide polymorphisms (SNPs) in TNF, LTA, and SLC11A1 genes and risk of endemic cutaneous leishmaniasis (CL) in Sri Lanka (Samaranayake et al., 2010). Comparison of the different ethnic groups showed the distribution of alleles of LTA+252 A>G to differ significantly in minority ethnic groups (Tamils and Moors) as compared to the majority ethnic group (Sinhalese). However, case-control studies did not reveal any association with occurrence of CL. Furthermore, variant allele distribution in other populations, where they are positively associated with leishmaniasis, differed significantly from the Sri Lankan group. Authors, therefore, suggested further investigations in to the association of human genetics with CL.

Samaranayake et al. (2016) studied HLA class I (HLA-A, HLA-B) and HLA class II (HLA-DRB1, HLADQB1) loci in cutaneous leishmaniasis in the Sinhalese, the major ethnic group in Sri Lanka. However, the study did not reveal any major association, except the fact that HLA-B locus was more polymorphic in the patients as compared to controls. Authors further mention that this study was restricted by inadequate sample numbers.

However, local study demonstrated high prevalence of HLA-B07 in controls, suggesting a protective tendency, and increased HLA B15 in patients, suggesting susceptibility. However, HLA Bw22, an allele similar to this has been identified as a risk factor and HLA B15 as a protective factor in the new world populations (Lara et al., 1991).

Sri Lankan studies on the human host have failed to draw major conclusions. The findings were not similar to those already available for other populations. Host genetic studies on leishmaniasis in the world are limited and have shown variable results. This may probably be due to the small number of studies including restricted sample sizes and conducted in geographically

separated populations in which baseline allele frequencies, parasite characteristics, and host responses may not be similar at all. Establishing a baseline data
for the local population with adequate coverage of all ethnic groups, properly
designed case-control studies with adequate sample size and inclusion of more
functional criteria such as SNP analyses and antigen expression are likely to
draw scientifically valid conclusions.

9.5 CONCLUSIONS

Many gaps still exist in the knowledge on immunopathology in Sri Lankan
leishmaniasis. *In situ* and systemic response patterns, their usefulness in
screening early and asymptomatic infection, monitoring disease progression
and predicting and assessing treatment response, and predicting disease outcomes and other functional relationships in relation to different disease phenotypes prevalent in the country would be useful for detection and control of
the disease. Furthermore, in-depth understanding of underlying mechanisms
leading to different immune-pathological sequelae would also be important.
Since the final clinical outcome is the result of ultimate balance between multiple factors, including host genetics, parasite genetics, host nutritional and
concurrent pathological status, it may not be easy to demonstrate the not so
strong associations unless other factors are controlled to keep the effect on the
outcome to a minimum or proper statistical measures are considered to counteract them during these studies. Associations between leishmaniasis and host
genetics will also be of importance to identify protective factors.

Enhanced Case Detection through Clinical and Laboratory Methods

10

Along with the scientific research on different aspects of the disease, improvements in the capacity in research and patient management are also important to achieve success in disease control. We have made several attempts on enhancing case detection, patient care, as well as on research. Other scientists and clinicians too have contributed in these areas. This chapter summarizes the work related to diagnostic aspects of leishmaniasis in Sri Lanka.

10.1 PLACE FOR CLINICAL DIAGNOSIS

Leishmania donovani are generally accepted as a species transmitted from human to human *via* the bite of a sandfly. Animal reservoirs that harbour *L. donovani* are not widely known except for a few reports in the recent past (El-Hassan et al., 1993; Hassan et al., 2009; Jambulingam et al., 2017). Therefore, timely case detection and early treatment with appropriate

DOI: 10.1201/9781003281801-10

anti-leishmanials is a main mode of disease control accepted by the WHO (2010). Enhanced clinical suspicion, confirmation through the use of locally appropriate laboratory tools, and timely, accurate, and complete case management with adequate follow-up are key points for success in controlling *L. donovani* infections in an endemic setting.

Self-referral is usually not immediate in leishmaniasis due to the non-disturbing nature of most initial lesions and lack of awareness. Making efforts for active case detection remains important.

Few attempts on active case detection surveys (Siriwardana et al., 2010; Kariyawasam et al., 2015; Ranasinghe et al., 2013), description of the clinical profile (many publications discussed in various chapters including Siriwardena et al., 2003; Rajapaksa et al., 2005; Siriwardana, 2008; Samaranayake et al., 2008; Nawaratna et al., 2007; Siriwardana et al., 2017), and development of a clinical scoring system (Siriwardana et al., 2015) and method comparison studies (Ranawaka et al., 2012; Ranasinghe et al., 2015; Kothalawala et al., 2016; de Silva et al., 2017) have been reported in the local setting to date.

Clinical detection of leishmaniasis is also challenging. None of the clinical markers are pathognomonic for any form of leishmaniasis. A variety of other dermatological conditions including lupus vulgaris, leprosy, and psoriasis are considered by clinicians in the differential diagnosis of leishmaniasis. Some locally developed guidelines are available for pharmacological management of cutaneous leishmaniasis (Karunaweera et al., 2013). However, the available treatment options are expensive and toxic. As such, preferably, cases need to be laboratory-confirmed prior to treatment. Accurate clinical suspicion, therefore, remains critical to enhance case confirmation.

Also, underreporting of diagnosed cases at clinical settings is a major concern in many leishmaniasis endemic settings, negatively affecting disease interventions and the global information base (Mosleh et al., 2008; Maia-Elkhoury et al., 2007; Copeland et al., 1990). Approximately only one-third of affected countries provide official notification to the WHO.

10.2 PATIENT-CENTRED COMMENCEMENT OF INTERVENTIONS

Furthermore, an understanding of early and late occurring clinical markers is also important since leishmaniasis can be slow-evolving with multiple clinical stages during its progression. Passive case detection (PCD) remains the mainstay of patient encounters in Sri Lanka at present, giving a very important place for the patient-centred commencement of interventions.

To facilitate this, attempts were made to develop a diagnostic clinical algorithm useful at the field and hospital level. Availability of a uniform set of clinical markers across an endemic area will, therefore, facilitate case screening, narrow down referrals for investigations, minimize unnecessary invasive procedures and investigation costs, and ensure a more accurate clinical diagnosis. Clinical markers are widely used in many clinical conditions (Ho et al., 2013; Davis et al., 2013; Ghosh et al., 2011; Diniz et al., 2011). However, clinical markers have not been well-described for leishmaniasis. Furthermore, generalizability of findings of small-scale studies is hindered by regional variation, which is a known barrier in leishmaniasis control (Stockdale et al., 2013). High degree of clinical suspicion is critical in leishmaniasis. Our study described for the first time a two-staged clinical algorithm that facilitates screening of cutaneous leishmaniasis in Sri Lanka by primary health care workers in stage 1 and management by medical professionals in stage 2.

Selected clinical markers of 400 patients suspected of cutaneous leishmaniasis were analysed retrospectively with laboratory confirmation of leishmaniasis. Ten clinical markers predicted cutaneous leishmaniasis with an over 90% accuracy. Subsets of markers showed high levels of sensitivities (60%–97.2%) and/or significant association with positive laboratory results as compared to negative lesions [typical onset (acne-form, painless non-itchy), ($P=0.026$), size up to 2 cm (P=0.046), well-defined edges (P=0.002), regular edges (P=0.018), rounded shape (P=0.030), and lesions at 5–8 months (P=0.052)]. Five of them (typical onset, number up to 2, small size, rounded edges, and rounded shape) also had >70% sensitivity levels as compared to laboratory findings. Typical onset had the highest sensitivity of 97% and a positive predictive value (PPV) of 72%. Lesions at 5–8 months duration having defined edges (P=0.013, specificity=89.7%, PPV=83.1) or having regular edges (P=0.006, specificity=86.2%, PPV=82.4%) were also predictive of cutaneous leishmaniasis. Most of early laboratory-confirmed (<12 months) lesions remained < 3cm in size (sensitivity > 67%, PPV > 70%) and had defined edges (sensitivity of 52%–71%, specificity of 46.7%–68.8%) (PPV of 75.1%–86%).

Four clinical markers served as good diagnostic markers in both early (≤4 months) and late (>12 months) lesions, namely, typical onset (91.3%–98.4%), presence of ≤2 lesions (sensitivity =82.6%–94.7%), size ≤2 cm (66.9%–73.7%), and regular edges (68.6%–76.3%). Reliability of clinical markers generally declined in chronic lesions. However, this study showed that clinical detection is not equally reliable in chronic lesions as compared to early lesions. Small lesions of over 12 months were highly indicative of cutaneous leishmaniasis (sensitivity of 66%, specificity of 66.7%). None of the single/combination markers, however, were 100% sensitive or specific, highlighting the undeniable usefulness of laboratory confirmation in diagnosis. Detailed understanding of local clinical presentations, increased case suspicion, and confirmation combined with establishment of good diagnostic tools are important.

Ranawaka et al. (2012) have also examined the reliability of clinical screening in the local setting. Both these studies have reported over 90% accuracy in the clinical diagnosis.

10.3 LABORATORY BASED METHODS

During the initial stages of the epidemic, laboratory diagnosis of leishmaniasis was carried out by simple light microscopic examination of the Giemsa-stained smears prepared from saline aspirations obtained from active edges of ulcers or margins of nodules and scrapings of lesions obtained using sterile scalpels. Second-line investigations (culture and PCR) were established later on.

Since adequate number of parasites is also a pre-requisite in most species-level studies and other studies, *in vitro* cultivation of *Leishmania* spp. is important.

10.4 *IN VITRO* PARASITE CULTURING

We attempted growing the parasites in our laboratory in Colombo with guidance from many established *Leishmania* laboratories overseas. London School of Tropical Medicine and Hygiene in UK, Laboratorie de Montpellier in France and Liverpool School of Tropical Medicine and Hygiene provided training to the author, experiment support, and valuable continued scientific inputs during the early stages.

Parasites from lesion material in some of the historical cases have been grown in traditional NNN medium mostly to achieve a transient parasite load sufficient to enable a microscopic diagnosis in smear-negative cases (Naotunne et al., 1990; Senevirathne et al., 1995). At the beginning of the epidemic, we were not well-equipped or technically knowledgeable to carry out *in vitro* cultures of *Leishmania*. Successful *in vitro* cultivation of the parasites of cutaneous leishmaniasis was carried out in the local laboratory using traditional Novy, McNeal and Nicolle (NNN) medium (Ihalamulla et al., 2002). Propagation of cultures in order to allow parasite multiplication required specific temperature maintenance between 22°C and 25°C, suitable medium, and strict sterile conditions. Sophisticated laboratory setups were required to achieve all these requirements, which significantly increased the cost of this technique.

As a solution, a simple clay device was designed and developed to maintain *Leishmania* cultures at low cost (Ihalamulla et al., 2004). A thermo-stable box-type clay device with a corrugated outer surface was made. Water was poured into the clay box and tubes containing parasite cultures were kept half-immersed in the water. Evaporation of water from the walls reduced the temperature in water within the pot, and adjustment of the water level allowed maintenance of temperature inside the clay device between 22°C and 25°C. This device enabled maintenance of parasite cultures in semi-solid media for a longer period of time. However, these attempts did not facilitate the mass cultures of the parasites.

Novy, McNeal, and Nicolle (NNN) medium and Evans' modified Tobie's medium, two conventional semi-solid media, were used in the laboratory for parasite isolation during initial stages. This was used mainly for patient diagnostic purposes. However, media preparation involved time-consuming and cumbersome procedures, parasite transformation and growth were slow, and mass cultures were not possible with semi-solid media. However, bulk culturing provided large numbers of parasites as a pre-requisite for our planned research projects. More simple and economical methods that avoid collection of rabbit blood, preparation of media, and use of glass tubes were required. Therefore, availability of a more sensitive technique with added advantages of being less cumbersome, quick to perform, and able to provide satisfactory results was required for this. Author's training in Liverpool School of Tropical Medicine and Hygiene in UK under the guidance of Dr. Michael Chance who was a pioneer researcher in establishing the gold-standard method of iso-enzyme characterization for *Leishmania* species identification allowed optimization of commercially available M199 culture medium for the local parasite for the growth of the Sri Lankan parasites. This enabled the establishment of mass cultivation techniques in Sri Lanka in 2004.

A simple study compared traditional bi-phasic media and liquid monophasic media for *Leishmania* cultivation with. Liquid monophasic medium was found less complex and less expensive and had better sensitivity (Ihalamulla et al., 2005).

With the commencement of our field-case detection activities, it was then necessary to maintain satisfactory rates of parasite culture positivity in spite of sample collections being carried out in the remote areas in Sri Lanka. Transport of clinical isolates to Colombo laboratory under sterile conditions and without much delay was difficult during field surveys. The journey took several hours. It was necessary to maintain temperature with the use of ice boxes, and often the samples arrived in Colombo at night, making it necessary for the technicians to work until late in the laboratory.

A simple culture technique that allowed both the use of monophasic culture medium and convenient inoculation in the field settings with high sensitivity was reported by a study group in Turkey (Allahverdiyev et al., 2004). A saline aspirate obtained from the skin lesions was mixed with equal volumes of monophasic RPMI culture medium, supplemented with 20% FCS, and microcapillary tubes were inoculated using the well-mixed solution, sealed with wax, and maintained at 23°C and 26°C in this method. This method was tested for its suitability for cultivation of Sri Lankan *Leishmania* parasites with encouraging results (Ihalamulla et al., 2005, 2006).

The microcapillary culture technique slowly replaced the use of SSM both in field and laboratory inoculations of *in vitro* cultures (unpublished data from author).

Cultivation of parasites can be carried out in many commercial media. A small-scale study was carried out to examine the suitability of M 199 commercial media, which was already optimized for mass cultures by that time. This study confirmed the suitability of M 199 supplemented with fetal calf serum for the use in capillary culture propagation (Ihalamulla et al., 2008). This technique is now being practiced for initial parasite isolation and routine diagnosis in our laboratory in Colombo.

Studies also examined the usefulness of microcapillary culture in long-distance transportation of live parasites (Ihalamulla et al., 2009). With increased case detection at field sites situated away from the central lab in Colombo, the ability to use this in long-distance transportation was a big advantage. Thus, the microcapillary method further ensured their suitability for field inoculation of samples and their convenient transport, allowing us to overcome a major obstacle.

Capillary cultures were transferred to large volume containers, and parasite cultures were slowly built up in to mass cultures over few weeks. *In vitro* culture of the parasites paves the way not only for diagnosis but for most of the research projects that required large numbers of parasites to date.

With the emergence of visceral leishmaniasis in Sri Lanka, scientists have made successful attempts in *in vitro* cultivation of visceralizing *Leishmania* parasites as well (Ranasinghe et al., 2012).

10.5 MOLECULAR METHODS

Diagnosis of leishmaniasis by molecular methods was identified as a useful alternative in smear and culture-negative isolates. Established PCR assays had been examined for the usefulness in the detection of *L. donovani* infection with successful results (Siriwardana, 2008; Ranasinghe et al., 2015; Kothalawala and Karunaweera 2016). Genus-specific mini-circle Kdna-based PCR using R221 and R332 primers (Lachaud et al., 2001) was used in the routine diagnosis of all microscopy and culture-negative samples since early stages of the Sri Lankan epidemic (Siriwardana, 2008).

Suitability of many *Leishmania* genus–specific primers, KDNA (Rodger et al., 1990; Salotra et al., 2001), and the LITS ITS1 region of *Leishmania* (El-Tai et al., 2000) has been examined with 71% sensitivity or with 92% sensitivity (Ranasinghe et al., 2015).

Loop-mediated isothermal amplification (LAMP) assay using established *Leishmania* genus–specific primers (Alam et al., 2011; Takagi et al., 2009) has been tested for local *Leishmania* detection with a sensitivity of 82.6% and a 100% specificity in comparison to light microscopy (Kothalawala et al., 2016). Positive and negative predictive values were 100% and 66%, respectively. Time and the cost of LAMP assay were approximately half of those of a nested PCR according to this study. LAMP testing is simple, field-friendly, inexpensive, and rapid with high reproducibility rates as compared to conventional PCR. However, the authors reported relatively low levels of sensitivity and negative predictive value when compared to microscopy or nested PCR.

10.6 IMMUNOLOGICAL ASSAYS

Immunological diagnostic methods have also been assessed. The diagnostic value of a new rapid diagnostic immune-chromatographic strip test (cutaneous leishmaniasis-Detect™ IC-RDT), that captures the peroxidoxin antigen of *Leishmania* amastigotes has been reported (de Silva et al., 2017). Only a minority (28.4%) of clinically suspected lesions had been detected by the new IC-RDT, while PCR detected 80% of such lesions. Specificity and PPV of both IC-RDT and SSS compared to those of PCR were 100%. The median parasite grading of the RDT-positive samples had been slightly higher than that of PCR-positive samples. The duration of the lesion was not associated with IC-RDT positivity.

Even though the focus of this paper is on the dianogstic suitability of the examined tool, low sensitivity obtained for local *Leishmania* infections with established RDT probably indicate the differences in the antigen profiles or differential expression of them in the local parasites. In fact, differences in the antigenic profiles between local and known *Leishmania* species were predicted from early stages. We attempted to develop an in-house ELISA to diagnose the local infections as explained in previous sections. According to the initial attempts, sero-prevalence of anti-*Leishmania* IgG antibodies in the study group was 34.0% (n = 17/50) (Siriwardana et al., 2018). The study was expanded to develop an in-house ELISA assay which enabled detection of a sero-prevalence of over 82% with 99.5% specificity (Deepachandi et al., 2020).

10.7 OPTIMAL AND IDEAL CASE DETECTION RATES

Leishmaniasis is characterized by the absence of characteristic clinical features, presence of complex presentations, and their geographical variation. Multiple approaches to achieve enhanced case suspicion remains crucial at all times. Periodic surveillance of clinical characteristics and trends in their presentations, vigilant identification of the occurrence of new clinical features in association with all forms of leishmaniasis, and dissemination of the growing knowledge in the research sector to clinical, preventive, and public sectors in appropriate proportions are required. A balance should be reached between the ideal target of detecting 100% cases within a minimal time and a more realistic target of detecting a decided proportion of cases within a defined time. These figures should be preferably decided by evidence and experience-based discussions between multisectoral stakeholders.

10.8 GAPS AND NEEDS

There are several obstacles in the journey towards achieving optimal case suspicion rates, though there are some formal pathways in dissemination of research knowledge into different sectors in the applied specialties in Sri Lanka. In the diagnosis of leishmaniasis, clinicians look for typical clinical manifestations or presentations. Atypical manifestations and asymptomatic cases receive minimal attention (Singh et al., 2014). There had been occasions where successive and detailed discussions had to be carried out with clinicians to draw their attention towards asymptomatic infection, when a *Leishmania* spp.–positive bone marrow report is made available for an apparently healthy individual, for a patient with a confirmed alternative diagnosis, for a patient with a positive microscopy report on a past leishmanial skin infection, for a person who recovers a minor febrile illness within 48–72 hours (author's personnel experience). This carries special importance in the local setting when atypical cutaneous leishmaniasis manifestations and micro changes within the existing cutaneous leishmaniasis profile and emergence of visceral leishmaniasis are observed. Many of our initial visceral leishmaniasis cases were investigated for leishmaniasis following a long list of other investigations performed to explore a series of other possibilities.

Long-lasting cutaneous leishmaniasis lesions are still presented to the clinical setting (Deepachandi et al., 2017), and some of them are first investigated over lengthy periods for alternative possibilities prior to consideration for leishmaniasis (authors unpublished observations).

Improved knowledge on clinical presentations coupled together with field-friendly inexpensive and accurate confirmatory diagnostic tests are important for Sri Lanka. This will minimize duration of illness, undesired sequelae of long-lasting illness, load of parasite reservoirs in the community, and socio-economic burden on the society as well. In addition to routine individual diagnosis, improved diagnostic tools can also empower disease burden estimation, studies on trends, and progression of infection as well, which are essential components of knowledge in designing disease control activities.

Diagnostic approaches that detect parasites remain the most specific tools available in the diagnosis of leishmaniasis. Microscopic examination of the lesion material in cutaneous leishmaniasis or muco-cutaneous leishmaniasis and bone marrow aspirates in visceral leishmaniasis are practiced as first-line diagnostic approaches in those respective clinical entities at present in Sri Lanka (Siriwardana et al., 2015, 2017; Rathnayake et al., 2010).

Sampling of lesions is carried out by trained technical officers or by medical professionals in the country. Also, bone marrow aspirations cannot be performed in the field settings. They have to be performed by specialist clinicians. The technique is painful, expensive, and associated with complications. Microscopy of such collected specimens does not allow higher sensitivities in spite of being highly specific. False-negative results are expected in chronic forms, atypical forms, and treated cases of cutaneous leishmaniasis. Often, newly appointed technical personnel are unable to detect parasites until they are taken through a series of several hundreds of *Leishmania*-positive slides (author's unpublished observations).

In vitro cultivation of parasites is limited to the Center for Leishmaniasis in the University of Colombo and few research laboratories in the country. All microscopy-negative patients had been offered a free of charge *in vitro* cultivation technique in the Colombo laboratory since the early stages of the epidemic. *In vitro* cultivation of lesion or organ aspirates has been shown to increase the sensitivity of microscopy to a great extent by allowing the parasites to grow in numbers (Maurya et al., 2010; Hide et al., 2007).

However, cultivation of *Leishmania* parasites demands many resources as mentioned already. Also, the sensitivity of culture tends to be low and highly variable (Faber et al., 2003). The microcapillary technique is used as a good alternative in various settings with a clearly improved detection rate (Pagheh et al., 2014).

Also, considering the high level of specificities, both tools evaluated by Kothalawala et al. (2016) and de Silva et al. (2017) could be used as second-line assays in microscopy-negative cases prior to proceeding with *in vitro* cultivation techniques.

Importantly, parasitological testing is the only confirmatory test which exists for relapsed patients.

Serological assay using the rK39 dipstick method is offered prior to invasive sample collections for parasitological confirmation to detect cases of visceral leishmaniasis on a routine basis in Colombo laboratory. There are various serological assays used in the diagnosis of leishmaniasis with varying sensitivity and specificity that depends on the antigen (and thus the antibody) of concern (Hasker et al., 2014). The rK39 negativity reported in previous local studies highlight the need for establishment of more locally appropriate tools. Service of a haematologist is not available in some main hospitals. Almost all other hospitals that handle large number of self-referrals in leishmaniasis are situated in main endemic areas in the North and South. Immunological tools will have the added advantage in visceral leishmaniasis detection, thus avoiding bone marrow aspirations.

In-house ELISA detected 82% of cutaneous leishmaniasis cases in Sri Lanka with provision for further development. This may be used at least in the initial screening of suspected cases with local *Leishmania* infection. This, however, has the limitations including the need of technical hands and laboratory facilities to perform.

PCR is offered in the Colombo laboratory for all microscopy and culture-negative clinically suspected cases of all forms of leishmaniasis, irrespective of whether they are included in research studies or not. However, the cost of investigation is a major drawback where provision of the facility depends on the availability of research funds. Diagnostic accuracy of molecular biological investigations is very high. However, their usefulness had been questioned on various occasions since they are not field-friendly. Only microscopy for cutaneous leishmaniasis diagnosis is available in the government sector hospitals at present.

All negative cases receive diagnostic confirmation at referral laboratories in a few Universities or proceed to treatment on clinical grounds at present (author's unpublished data).

10.9 CONCLUSIONS

Research on field-friendly and locally suitable diagnostic tools is a timely requirement. Low cost and simple procedures will be an added advantage in a developing country. Once established, decentralization of the facilities, allocation of resources, and training laboratory personnel will ensure good case detection.

Treatment Methods

11

Early, accurate, and complete treatment of leishmaniasis is important to cure the illness and prevent negative sequelae of long-standing illness on the patient and community. Early treatment of all forms of leishmaniasis can theoretically reduce the parasite reservoirs in the community, though asymptomatic infections are not treated at present.

11.1 CHOICE BETWEEN SELF-CURE AND INTERVENTION

Leishmanial infections are treated based on the nature of clinical outcome, sequelae, and complications. These factors are known to depend on the causative species or subspecies of *Leishmania* mainly owing to the different levels of parasite virulence and host genetics.

In Sri Lanka, whether skin lesions induced by *Leishmania donovani* should be treated or should be left for self-cure is still uncertain. Considering the causative species being originally a visceralizing parasite, classical skin lesions may self-heal or disseminate to distant mucosal or visceral sites in long-standing infections. However, follow-up studies carried out on cutaneous leishmaniasis have not shown visceralization (Kariyawasam et al., 2017), while cutaneous leishmaniasis is associated with a high sero-prevalence (Deepachandi et al., 2020 and Siriwardana et al., 2018). Unresolved long-standing infections progressing to full-blown ulceration or persistent nodular stages are not uncommon (author's personal observations). Adequate treatment in cutaneous leishmaniasis is recommended in order to prevent or minimize complications and undesired outcomes of long-standing infection if uneventful self-recovery is not the expected outcome. Main indications for treatment in classical cutaneous leishmaniasis include the need to accelerate healing in disseminated disease or chronic disease, leading to disfiguring

DOI: 10.1201/9781003281801-11

ulcers and subsequent scars (*L. major*) and involvement of sensitive areas (e.g., lesions over face or adjacent to mucosal tissue, genitalia, or over the joints). Some other indications are cutaneous leishmaniasis including *Leishmania recidivans*, primary cutaneous leishmaniasis leading to mucosal leishmaniasis with possibility of secondary mucosal infection, (e.g., *Leishmania viannia subgenus*), possibility of visceralization (e.g., *L. donovani* causing CL), infection in non-immune travellers, and when the causative species is unknown. Shortening the course of illness and therefore prevention of local and systemic dissemination, disfigurement, psycho-social disturbances, and reduction of the cost of the illness are expected by active intervention in CL. Clinically apparent visceral leishmaniasis and muco-cutaneous leishmaniasis always require timely and complete treatment. Treatment options in leishmaniasis are selected based on the severity and extent of morbidity and risk of mortality associated with the various disease forms.

Treatment response is also known to depend on the parasite species (Allen et al., 1989; Navin et al., 1992; Hadighi et al., 2006). This has been examined in a few studies conducted in Sri Lanka. *L. donovani* are known to be more sensitive to anti-leishmanial therapy as compared to skin localizing species (*Leishmania major*, *L. tropica*, and *L. mexicana*) (Allen et al., 1989). In addition to the species, the final outcome of treatment is determined by multiple factors related to the drug pharmacokinetics and usage (mechanisms of action, protocol used, delivery techniques, and level of adherence to treatment) and patient factors (immunity, co-illnesses, clinical parameters of the lesion such as duration, level of enlargement, multiplication, and location) (Chakravarty et al., 2010; Sundar et al., 1994).

Therefore, the outcome of genetically different *L. donovani* causing skin infection cannot be easily predicted without proper scientific evidence. Decision-making on whether to leave a lesion for self-cure or to treat with expensive and toxic anti-leishmanials is important.

Information on treatment outcome in *L. donovani*–induced cutaneous leishmaniasis are scarce in global literature. WHO guidelines are also based on those traditionally cutaneous leishmaniasis causing *Leishmania* species. Therefore, it is very important for Sri Lanka to establish treatment practices based on locally obtained scientific evidence.

11.2 LOCALLY AVAILABLE OPTIONS

At the onset of the recent epidemic of leishmaniasis, Sri Lanka was ill-equipped with regard to case detection and management. Cryotherapy which is a treatment method used for many dermatological conditions was the first treatment measure practiced. In a preliminary observation carried out at the onset of the epidemic, lesions of cutaneous leishmaniasis improved with multiple sessions of cryotherapy (Siriwardana et al., 2003). However, repeated hospital visits and minor side effects were observed. Cryotherapy is not a recommended anti-leishmanial treatment option. Due to its wider availability, this inexpensive and easy-to-administer treatment was commonly practiced at the few major hospitals where cases of leishmaniasis were detected. Leaving for self-cure was not the practice mainly due to the potentially dangerous nature of the causative parasite species.

Soon after, treatment of cutaneous leishmaniasis with sodium stibogluconate replaced treatment with cryotherapy in most clinical settings. SSG was administered either intra-lesionally in single lesions or intra-muscularly in multiple or facial lesions. Every other day, weekly or fortnightly regimens of SSG and weekly or fortnightly regimens of cryotherapy have been the practice at different dermatological clinics. Sodium stibo-gluconate (SSG) injections given through intra-lesional or intra-muscular route and cryotherapy are the commonly practiced treatment options for cutaneous leishmaniasis in Sri Lanka. Limited number of cases of visceral leishmaniasis have been successfully treated with intra-venous SSG, amphotericin, or oral miltefosine without poor response or subsequent recurrences at 3-year follow-up (Siriwardana et al., 2017).

However, it is necessary to understand the benefits and outcomes of each of these regimes through properly designed clinical trials with adequate follow-up durations. Currently available research output on treatment options is very limited in this country. Locally available cheap and easy-to-use treatment options (cryotherapy, hypertonic saline, and thermotherapy) have been explored in comparison to SSG treatment at few occasions.

First such study was reported in 2010 by Ranawaka et al. Hypertonic saline had been tested and reported to be effective for local patient populations with cutaneous leishmaniasis (Ranawaka et al., 2010). Efficacy and safety of intra-lesional 7% hypertonic saline in comparison to intra-lesional SSG showed a 100% cure rate with one to six injections (average 3.24). Hypertonic saline has shown a slightly less (92.2%) cure rate which required 1–10 injections (average 5.27). Average duration of treatment with SSG was slightly less than that of HS (5.11 and 8.78 weeks). None of these treatment options have shown to depend on the clinical type, size, duration, or affected bodily site of the lesions. Local or systemic side effects have not been observed except for pain during injection. This group was followed up for a period of 18 months. Recurrence or visceralization was not observed during the follow-up period.

Efficacy of intra-lesional liquid nitrogen treatment (cryotherapy) in local cutaneous leishmaniasis has also been examined with encouraging results

(Ranawaka et al., 2011). A total of 91.7% of patients were cured within a mean number of 3.5 (1–4) cryotherapy sessions. Increased cure rates were demonstrated for early smaller (<1 cm) lesions and head and upper limb lesions when compared to rates observed for lesions in lower limbs (71.42%) and trunk (66.66%). Side effects were minor, including ulceration (33%), depigmentation (46.9%), and scarring (43%). During 6 months of follow-up, there was one (1.6%) recurrence. The authors recommended fortnightly application of cryotherapy for smaller lesions, avoiding the face, and on patients who have a tendency to form keloids.

Intra-lesional 7% hypertonic saline (HS) has been shown to be effective and safe against cutaneous leishmaniasis caused by *L. donovani* and *L. major*, with cure rates of 92% and 96%, respectively. This study was designed to assess the efficacy and safety of 10% and 15% HS in CL. The follow-up period was 18 months. High cure rates were observed for both 10% HS (93%) and 15% HS (93.6%) preparations with mean 3.6 (1–10) injections and 5.28 (2–10) injections, respectively. Treatment with 10% HS was completed within 6 weeks, while that with 15% HS required 9 weeks.

Thermotherapy had been tested for its efficacy, safety, and cost-effectiveness on locally acquired cutaneous leishmaniasis with single lesions (Refai et al., 2017). A group of 98 patients receiving single sessions of radiofrequency-induced heat therapy (RFHT) at 50°C for 30 seconds had achieved a 66% cure rate at the end of a year without major adverse effects as compared to 59.4% cure rate achieved with IL-SSG treatment. Cost of treatment was assessed using the scenario building technique. The cure rate achieved by RFHT was significantly higher than the cure rate of SSG treatment during early weeks but was comparable after 10 weeks. Authors have reported a single application of RFHT as a safe, cost-effective, and convenient option as compared to multiple doses of IL-SSG for treatment of cutaneous leishmaniasis in Sri Lanka.

11.3 POOR RESPONSE AND DRUG RESISTANCE

In the meantime, treatment failure or delayed response in local lesions of cutaneous leishmaniasis with standard therapy were reported from different dermatology clinics (author's personal communications, Refai et al., 2016).

Atypical lesions in cutaneous leishmaniasis have shown to require treatment with SSG over longer periods when compared to the regimen of the same drug required to achieve a clinical cure in classical lesions in cutaneous disease (Siriwardana et al., 2019).

Observation of poor response to standard anti-leishmanials in Sri Lanka further indicate the necessity for carefully selected treatment protocols for these drugs in Sri Lanka. Drug resistance in leishmaniasis is an increasingly reported problem throughout the world (Roychoudhury et al., 2008). The selection should be based on accurately carried out treatment trials. Once the selections are carried out, continued surveillance for their efficacy should be maintained. The current observation also predicts the future need for effective alternative options. Added advantages of such a solution would be low cost, availability, and ability to store and administer easily.

Patient compliance can be enhanced with a reduced number of hospital visits and minimal or absent side effects of the selected treatment option.

Careful monitoring of emergence of drug resistance is also required. Wrong practices had been the base for emergence of drug resistance in many endemic settings (Chakravarty et al., 2010; Lira et al., 1999; Allen et al., 1989). Recently observed good response rates to anti-leishmanials in visceral leishmaniasis in the local setting is encouraging. Unavailability of the drugs at clinical settings, poor compliance, and lack of a system for active tracing of drop outs could lead to establishment of drug resistance in Sri Lanka.

Capacity Building, A Model for Handling Emerging Health Issues

12

12.1 RATIONAL THINKING, STEPWISE APPROACH, AND PERSISTENCE IN DEVELOPMENT

Following the detection of a single case of leishmaniasis in 2001, while the clinicians look forward to providing treatment, it was necessary for us as scientists to focus on a different aspect. We were left with multiple questions and challenges. Colombo laboratory, as a University establishment, therefore, adopted a multifaceted approach including raising community awareness, providing patient care, establishing diagnostic facilities, initiating essential research, training different categories in healthcare and research, and establishment of necessary infra- structure for all these activities. This chapter outlines the different activities carried out at different points in time with a view to enabling the young scientists take a rational approach towards similar encounters including other emerging issues in different settings in future. Later on, many other local

DOI: 10.1201/9781003281801-12

research institutions also have carried out research to enrich the scientific database with valuable information. Authorities including the Ministry of Healthcare and Nutrition have come forward to initiate necessary action.

Upon detection of local occurrence of even a single case of a disease that is new to a community, first it is rational to attempt at discovering the hidden true burden of the same. Case identification, provision of patient care, and commencement of research were immediately felt other needs with regard to the problem at hand. Since the characteristics of leishmaniasis are known to be complex and differ between endemic settings, it was specially required to obtain essential local information through scientific approaches. Key scientific question that needed to be answered immediately following this laboratory report was where did this patient acquire leishmaniasis and if there is local transmission, where were the other cases?

12.2 INITIAL ATTEMPTS IN AWARENESS RAISING

In order to discover the hidden reservoir of cases and answer these questions, the first step has to be raising awareness among the professionals and general public. Since the index patient probably acquired infection while at work in Weli-Oya, a war-affected area in Northern Sri Lanka, an awareness seminar was held for the professionals at the Victory Hospital in Anuradhapura, the main healthcare institution receiving army referrals from the patient's location. Over 12 other awareness campaigns were also held by the author immediately afterward for medical, para-medical, and general public sectors in war-affected borderline areas in this area under military cover. Programmes covered the district hospital, schools, home guard officers, military and police officers, and civilians in these areas. Accurate selection of target groups and timing of awareness programmes were two key things for success.

These were only decided after gathering information from patients coming to Colombo, personal visits of the author to this area, and discussions carried out with then Brigade commander and his officials in the army camp in the area. Awareness activities resulted in a snowballing effect in knowledge dissemination, resulting in increased self-referrals and emergence of volunteering community leaders. Meanwhile, when case reporting started from the South along with the transfer of the dermatologist who was serving the main health care institution that referred the index case (general hospital, Anuradhapura) to a major hospital in the region, awareness programmes were extended to Southern Sri Lanka. Our target groups were civilians, para-medical personnel, and medical professionals in this area. We were able to detect many more cases within first 12 months, confirming the presence of an already established and widespread local transmission of leishmaniasis within the island.

12.3 INITIAL ATTEMPTS IN PATIENT CARE

A leishmaniasis diagnostic laboratory was established following the detection of the first few cases in the Department of Parasitology of Faculty of Medicine that offered clinical evaluation and light microscopy for diagnosis on a weekly basis. This clinic was held every Tuesday to fall in line with the dermatology clinic held at National Hospital in Colombo, just across the road. Patients clinically screened at places in the North were referred to this dermatology clinic. They were investigated on the same day in our laboratory, and a report was provided before the next clinic visit during which they underwent liquid nitrogen treatment upon laboratory confirmation of CL. The country was ill-equipped to handle cases of leishmaniasis during that time. Liquid nitrogen therapy was the only available treatment option. Patients were offered a free-of-charge follow-up facility for a period of 2 years at the author's institution.

However, patients presenting from the North had to pass through over six stations (peripheral and central health care settings and army camps), spending few days to visit the author's institution for a simple diagnostic report. Therefore, discussions were carried out by the author with military officials in North and a direct referral system from peripheral army camps to the University was established.

Meanwhile, educational material was also developed and awareness campaigns were extended to cover more areas in the North and South. By the end of the first 24 months, 114 patients from 14/25 districts had been diagnosed by us. Soon after, the University clinic and the laboratory was serving the whole country and provided free-of-charge laboratory diagnosis through microscopy and a free follow-up facility.

12.4 INITIAL ATTEMPTS IN RESEARCH

With the increasing numbers of patients, the first formal clinical study was also commenced in year 2001, despite very limited resources. The clinical study did not require much funding. However, financial resources are an essential component for progression of any research programme. The first application made to the local National Science Foundation for a financial grant received due attention. It was selected for funding which eventually enabled maintenance of the laboratory and clinical services offered by us.

It was then necessary to establish more sensitive diagnostic tools for patient detection. However, the local laboratory was not equipped to handle this situation. Support and guidance were therefore sought from established overseas laboratories, namely, Laboratoire de Montpellier in France and Liverpool School of Tropical Medicine and Hygiene in UK through a doctoral scholarship award received by the author. This enabled eventual establishment of patient diagnosis by *in vitro* cultivation and PCR techniques. Successful cultivation of *Leishmania* parasites also led to the isolation of adequate parasite material that was necessary for many research techniques.

12.5 THE NEED FOR ENHANCED CAPACITY

With continued case reporting, it was necessary to further enhance case detection, case management, and research activities. Enhancement of capacity in whatever discipline involves a few key elements. It is important to accurately identify the priority areas for action to discriminate between essential and non-priority research interests and physical resources, approaching correct resources for funding, expertise, and persistence in these attempts until the targets are achieved.

12.6 DEVELOPING CAPACITY IN PATIENT CARE AND RESEARCH

12.6.1 Expertise

Along with the continued case reporting in Sri Lanka, expanding the dimensions of research and establishment of more sensitive diagnostic tools in clinical settings became our urgent requirements. The country was ill-equipped with regard to expertise and physical resources in achieving these targets. Established, trusted, and continued relationships with content experts are indispensable in such activities. Collaboration and guidance received from many overseas experts on leishmaniasis have significantly improved our capacity.

In addition to the advice and support received *via* online routes, The World Academy of Sciences (TWAS) science exchange programme and availability of research funds and training through Commonwealth scholarships, World Health Organization (WHO), and National Institute of Health in USA (NIH/USA) have enabled the visits of several experts to the local laboratory. Establishment of many essential techniques including an *in vivo* animal model for *Leishmania* propagation, improvements in mass cultivation techniques, immunological techniques, and many other experiments were established through these programmes. In addition, one-to-one meetings with research trainees, discussions with regard to their own research ideas, and outputs were also facilitated. Participation at overseas training programmes and scientific conferences by our team members have also been useful in capacity building.

12.6.2 Funds

Access to funding resources constitute an essential part in developing the capacity. Funding applications should be carefully designed with proper justification especially when such an application is made for investigating an emerging illness. Funding authorities need to be first convinced with regard to the usefulness of their investments on a project on an emerging issue. In addition, research activities per se do not constitute the whole requirement during the developmental stage of a laboratory. Building the physical infrastructure, developing the capacity of personnel, and increasing the visibility are equally important. Financial back up from local and overseas funding bodies including University Grants Commission, Commonwealth Scholarship Association, World Health Organization, and more recently University of Colombo and National Institute of Health, USA have supported these activities up to date.

12.6.3 Physical Setting

The weekly patient clinic has now expanded as the centre for leishmaniasis research, training, and diagnosis of UCFM. Activities take place in the three main lines described above. Scaling up of facilities to suit the increasing demands should preferably be carried out while targeting a maximum output, optimum utilization, and minimal wastage of resources. This is an important point specially for an institution located in a developing country.

12.6.4 Connectivity

Connecting with the external resources and enabling others to connect with us when required are always mutually beneficial. This is especially important during the development stages as it enables inter-laboratory or inter-country sharing of knowledge, skills, and attitudes. The website of the centre was established with a view to improve our visibility, adoption, to disseminate information, and to advertise our services. This includes essential information to the general public, healthcare staff, and undergraduate and post-graduate trainees. This also acts as a resource to acquire more information and details of the services available (https://med.cmb.ac.lk/parasitology/pdru/leishmaniasis/ctrdl/).

12.7 IMPACT ON SOCIETY AND HEALTHCARE DELIVERY

12.7.1 An Action Plan

Once the knowledge base is developed up to a satisfactory level, at least to include essential basic information to draw up a disease control plan for a country, the researcher's next responsibility would be the dissemination of such knowledge through proper channels at a proper time and motivating, guiding, and supporting their fellow scientists for necessary action. A model action plan is given here (Figure 12.1). In 2009, an international colloquium was convened by the University of Colombo in Collaboration with the Ministry of Healthcare and Nutrition. This conference was attended by many international content experts and local stakeholders. An action plan for leishmaniasis control in Sri Lanka was developed at this conference. The findings of the author's first formal study were useful in the development of a scientific platform for immediate, medium-, and long-term activities. Further to the action plan, national treatment guidelines were developed by the dermatologists in Sri Lanka. Leishmaniasis was also declared a notifiable disease in Sri Lanka as immediate follow-up action.

Periodic evaluation and reflection constitute an important part of our action. A second international colloquium was held 4 years later in 2013, with a wider international participation to review the first action plan.

Improving the ability of the team members to carry out different tasks with efficiency is important. This first included training technical officers for microscopic diagnosis. At the beginning, our technical officers were inexperienced

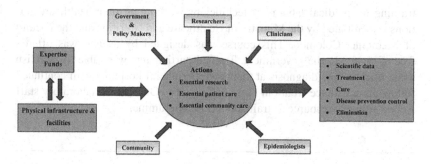

FIGURE 12.1 Model action plan.

in investigating patients for leishmaniasis, except for focusing few fixed smears containing plenty of typical *Leishmania* spp. amastigote forms under oil emersion lenses during undergraduate teaching sessions. Therefore, training them for routine diagnosis was an essential part of the work. Routine exercise, close supervision, and continued communication with experts and visiting scientist programmes have been useful in this. When the technical expertise was developed over many years in this way, they started serving as resource persons for our trainees and junior technicians.

In the meantime, technical staff was trained to perform PCR, culturing, and other techniques to facilitate routine diagnosis. Different categories of permanent, research, or temporary staff members of the department or outsiders visiting the department have been trained on the techniques necessary for both routine diagnosis and research. These include training of other categories (research students, routine assistants of the department, temporary trainees sent through other institutions, laboratory attendants, etc.).

12.8 CAPACITY BUILDING IN OTHER STAKEHOLDER SECTORS

Once the laboratory is self-sufficient, it is important to take necessary action to train others and decentralize the services. This helps in developing even a larger team for support in achieving desired targets. The country was facing diagnostic difficulties due to lack of trained persons. This increased the number of patients investigated by our centre in Colombo in thousands. Therefore, at the second international colloquium on leishmaniasis, we proposed that formal training on laboratory diagnosis is given to all government laboratory technicians (medical or public health). As a result, formal leishmaniasis training for medical laboratory technicians working at main healthcare stations was initiated by the Ministry of Healthcare and Nutrition and the Faculty of Medicine, Colombo. This course was designed by us and was offered free of charge to the government. Trained participants were able to establish basic microscopic diagnosis at their own peripheral hospitals with continued follow-up assistance from our team in Colombo. Our trained laboratory staff were a valuable resource as trainers in this programme.

12.9 PROFESSIONAL AWARENESS

In addition to the *ad hoc* awareness programmes, more formal and routinely carried out knowledge dissemination can be a better long-term investment. Leishmaniasis was introduced to the curricula of government public health laboratory technicians in the country. This was an important group in the Sri Lankan healthcare system, with high potential for expansion. They are currently involved in the laboratory diagnosis of leishmaniasis. In addition, undergraduate and post-graduate medical trainees of many specialties receive inputs on global and local situation of leishmaniasis at present.

12.10 PLANNING FOR SCALABILITY, VISIBILITY, AND ADOPTION

Useful lessons learnt through all these activities should preferably be added to increase the visibility and adoption of a laboratory. Further developments in research and research capacity should pave the way for a re-look at the national action plan, probably leading to the requests to include Sri Lanka in regional efforts in leishmaniasis elimination.

12.11 TEAM BUILDING

Team efforts are always essential in achieving such targets. Both enthusiasm and capabilities of team members form the pillars for success. During the first decade, the work was carried out by myself, a single technical officer and a single laboratory attendant with support and guidance from the head and staff of department. Short-term temporary staff have contributed to handling patients at times. Preferred composition of the team can change along with the changing trends of the research problem concerned. Later on, statisticians, molecular biologists, immunologists, epidemiologists, haematologists, and physicians have contributed to our research work immensely. The team has grown up from three members (2002) to over 16 internal members and many local and international collaborators today (2021).

Once the foundation of an establishment is complete, periodic assessment of the structure and activities, reflection, and improvements in main input lines (funding, expert assistance, infrastructure) and main output lines (research information, our tools and our services) is important.

Gaps in Knowledge, Current and Future Needs

13

13.1 SOUTH EAST ASIA REGION, INFORMATION GAPS AND NEEDS

Scientists have already pointed towards the potential issues related to the complex nature of the taxonomically divergent *Leishmania* parasites prevalent in the Asian region (Chang et al., 2018).

Valuable lessons in combatting leishmaniasis are available from the neighbourhood of Sri Lanka. Many countries in the SEA region report leishmaniasis at present (Bangladesh, Bhutan, India, Nepal, Sri Lanka, and Thailand) (Alvar et al., 2012). India, Nepal, and Bangladesh are known to be highly endemic for leishmaniasis since long, while Sri Lanka, Bhutan, and Thailand have reported leishmaniasis fairly recently. All six countries report visceral leishmaniasis. In addition, India and Sri Lanka have cutaneous leishmaniasis transmission as well (Alvar et al., 2012). The value in studying different epidemiological types prevalent in the Asian region has been highlighted (Chang et al., 2018).

In 2005, a regional kala-azar elimination initiative was launched in India, Nepal, and Bangladesh. This programme first aimed at reducing case numbers so that leishmaniasis is no longer considered a public health problem by reducing the numbers to a level of less than one per 10,000 population at the district level in Nepal and at the sub-district level in Bangladesh and in India (WHO, 2005). The used strategy mainly focused on early diagnosis, complete treatment, and integrated vector management (WHO, 2014). This programme faced many difficulties during its implementation and initially failed to achieve its targets. It was subsequently extended from 2015 to 2017 (WHO, 2014). Few years later in 2012, the WHO roadmap was drawn with a view to eliminate leishmaniasis from the region by year 2020. Very impressive progress was demonstrated by India, Nepal, and Bangladesh over the past few years by significantly reducing the incidence of new cases in all three countries by year 2015 (by around 67% in Bangladesh, 61% in India, and 46% in Nepal), (Chowdhury et al., 2014; Gurunath et al., 2014). Availability of point-of-care diagnostics and treatment at government primary healthcare level and reduction of transmission through vector control have been key interventions in this regard (Matlashewski et al., 2014).

Along with this not so easy pathway towards the achievements, several temporary failures too have been reported. These include failures in vector control efforts, resistance to first-line antimony therapy, high cost of treatment, and limited access to alternative options (Muniaraj, 2014; Chowdhury et al., 2014; Bhandari et al., 2011). There were several key determinants of success in these countries. They were the anthroponotic nature in disease transmission without animal involvement, absence of diversity in vector species and their susceptibility to existing insecticides, clear spatial demarcation in disease transmission areas, and availability of rapid diagnostic kits for diagnosis and availability of oral miltefosine for treatment (Bhattacharya et al., 2006)

Thailand and Bhutan reported low incidence of leishmaniasis and report only sporadic cases. However, the two countries joined with Nepal, Bangladesh, and India in efforts to eliminate leishmaniasis by 2017 in their countries (WHO, 2014). In spite of these efforts and outcomes, mathematical modelling, however, predicts continued *Leishmania donovani* transmission even after 2020 in this region (Le Rutte et al., 2017). Careful surveillance and assessment of the efficacy of control measures are of utmost significance in this region.

However, predictions suggest that *L. donovani* transmission will continue in the Indian sub-continent even after year 2020, necessitating a careful surveillance and control (Le Rutte et al., 2017).

However, as the incidence of VL declines towards the elimination goal, greater targeting of control methods will be required to ensure appropriate early action to prevent the resurgence of VL. Priorities are on surveillance to prevent resurgence with increased susceptibility of less immune individuals, implement modified control methods, and develop diagnostics and treatment options. History has shown periodic resurgence of leishmaniasis in 15-year cycles in India. PKDL and VL-HIV co-infection are posing threats to disease elimination by harbouring parasite reservoirs (Hirve et al., 2017; Gedda et al., 2020; Sundar et al., 2018; Rijal et al., 2019). Emergence of sub-populations of *L. donovani*, genetic exchanges, and mutations and complexities in response to drug treatment are already reported challenges in the period of surveillance (Imamura et al., 2016; Cuypers et al., 2018).

Factors that determine disease propagation in the community are studied (Chakravarty et al., 2019; Das et al., 2020).

13.2 SITUATION IN SRI LANKA

Nearly two decades have elapsed since the detection of the current epidemic in Sri Lanka. This focus that harbours the world's largest epidemic of dermotropic *L. donovani* with recent emergence of other clinical forms is not yet a part of this regional drive. Emergence of new genetic variants of *L. donovani*, of which some are dermotropic in the same region, requires more attention. Leishmaniasis in Sri Lanka and in Kerala in India represent two nearly similar problems (Siriwardana et al., 2003; Kumar et al., 2015). *L. donovani*–induced skin infections and other unusual clinical forms is a field that require increased attention (Thakur et al., 2018).

Epidemic of leishmaniasis occurring in Sri Lanka presents many unique characteristics. Presence of an unusual parasite, changing clinical presentations, and the many complexities associated with cutaneous leishmaniasis are some of them. These findings present many challenges in patient care and disease control. Variant parasites can result in many unforeseen sequalae that include unusual clinical outcomes , variations in treatment response and disease transmission characteristics. This indicates the necessity for designing disease control strategies after careful evaluation of all these.

Preliminary evidence for presence of potential animal reservoirs, diversity of vector species, potential to develop insecticide resistance, widespread geographical distribution of cases and lack of efficient field detection methods, and poor treatment response patterns can pose major challenges to local disease control efforts. The on-going COVID-19 pandemic might also affect negatively by further delaying case referrals and general diversion of common resources and infrastructure towards it.

Though a considerable amount of information is now available, many gaps still exist in the description and aetiology of the existing problem and identification of best suited interventional strategies and methods for implementation of them. Both basic and applied research is required to fill in such gaps. Definition of such local research priorities, establishment of more formal systems for research and application of resultant knowledge in practice, and strengthened, monitored, and continued operation of interventions will be the key steps in leishmaniasis control in an endemic setting.

13.3 LOCAL RESEARCH NEEDS

Multiple priority areas can be identified with regard to patient care and disease control. Clinical profile and its changing trends, treatment outcome and determining factors, establishment of infection in host, disease transmission in community, and vector and reservoir studies need to be continued. Similarly, an insight into still unthought-of or unpredicted scientific issues and active probing to see whether such problems exist would be equally important. Emergence of visceral leishmaniasis, presence of atypical clinical presentations, asymptomatic infection in the community, a higher than reported disease burden, different immunological response patterns, and presence of separate independent disease foci within the country are some of them which we predicted through informal observations earlier (Siriwardana et al., 2017, 2018, 2019). The young researcher will certainly discover more problems if careful attention is given to the changing trends of leishmaniasis in the local setting.

Identification of all infections and elimination of the parasite reservoir would theoretically be the ideal in controlling *L. donovani* infection. Occurrence of asymptomatic infection is considered to be ten times higher than that of the clinically apparent infections (Singh et al., 2014). Lengthy and variable incubation periods, occurrence of atypical clinical manifestations, lack of pathognomonic clinical features, complexity and instability and changing profiles of clinical presentations, and low awareness levels in professional and public sectors unfortunately lead to poor rates of case detection. Description of clinical profiles and changing trends have been carried out to a considerable extent in the country. However, lack of awareness among the public sector and even in the clinical settings, especially on the emergence of new clinical forms and occurrence of unusual forms and changing trends, still exist to a considerable degree (author's observations). One way to counteract this complex clinical picture is periodic clinical surveillance and raising awareness among those at-risk groups and treating clinicians.

Possibility of PKDL in local visceral leishmaniasis is not yet known. If present, this would present yet another important area of silent parasite reservoirs to be addressed. Meanwhile, all affected individuals may not seek treatment due to their less apparent clinical infection.

Availability of sensitive and reliable diagnostic tools is important. Laboratory investigations allow confirmation of patients who require treatment and minimize the chances of other clinically similar conditions receiving expensive and toxic anti-leishmanials. The value of PCR-based molecular diagnostic methods for detection of infection, relapse, and poor response in leishmaniasis have been highlighted due to poor performance of serological assays in discriminating these conditions (Sundar et al., 2018). The target product profile of a point-of-care diagnostic tool for cutaneous leishmaniasis include field-friendly, economical tools that enable case and follow up investigations (Cruz et al., 2019). Inexpensive and field-friendly nature of such tools and the ability to detect asymptomatic cases are definite added advantages.

At present, light microscopy for cutaneous lesions is effectively carried out at many peripheral hospital settings by the technical personnel trained at our institution. This has resulted in a significant reduction in the patient inflow to Colombo laboratory. For detection of VL, it is, however, necessary to depend on bone marrow aspiration. Non-invasive yet effective methods to detect all three forms of leishmaniasis would be of great importance.

It is encouraging to note that recently emerged cases of visceral leishmaniasis have responded well to currently available antimony compounds in spite of reports of poor response among cases of CL. However, the most challenging issue would be the prevention or delaying the emergence of drug resistance in the country. Evidence-based selection and careful use of treatment modalities are very important especially with the emergence of poor treatment response in cutaneous leishmaniasis. Local examination of new options including physical methods (for CL, non-pharmacological) and indigenous methods of treatment backed up by long-term and adequate follow up to look for resistance and recurrence will be some challenges facing the new researcher. The need for attending to patient perspectives such as quality of life, recurrence, and sterile cure, scar formation, stigmatization, and disability in CL drug trial design is now recommended (Erber et al., 2020).

Vector research including vector incrimination, behaviours, spatial and temporal distribution, insecticide susceptibility, search on animal reservoirs including types, distribution and transmission dynamics including environmental, socio-demographical, and behavioural factors is all important areas that require continued study. Effectiveness of vector control activities needs to be kept under surveillance, once implemented. In the absence of a suitable parasite antigen–based methods, tools that detect the level of population exposure to sandfly vectors will be of importance.

Clustering of cases in well-defined geographical locations in endemic countries in the ISC has been considered an advantage in control efforts. However, in Sri Lanka, there is widespread cases, though total geographical area is smaller than that in India. Identification of those factors enabling case clustering and emergence of hot spots through island wide active case detection programme is a timely need.

It is possible that three different strains of *L. donovani*, that is, visceralizing strains causing classical visceral leishmaniasis, non-visceralizing strains causing classical cutaneous infection, and a group of dermotropic strains causing non-classical viscerotropic leishmaniasis exist in the country. A clear understanding of why and how dermotropic parasites remain so, why and how the visceralizing proportion of parasites behave so, underlying immune pathological sequelae, and operationally useful markers that emerge from these various processes are of importance.

13.4 WAY FORWARD

Prioritization of research areas can be economical in a developing country while it allows the local researcher to stay more focused and obtain locally relevant information in a timely manner. Careful thinking and a genuine interest of the emerging local researcher undoubtedly has the power to bring about significant changes in a society. This is especially important to our own setting. An opportunity full of very special, interesting, and unique but yet unanswered research questions is just awaiting their attention.

Once the findings are made available, the researcher holds a very important role in knowledge dissemination to the relevant authorities at the correct time and using the most suitable approach. Sri Lanka is already blessed with many strengths that are necessary to handle this situation. Sri Lanka has a well-established and efficient health care infrastructure in place. Also, there are many other formal pathways for dissemination of information. The Ministry of Healthcare and Nutrition conducts regular meetings with almost all professional colleges in the field of medicine. The National Committee on Communicable Diseases which include members from research community as well is an authority that handles many important health care issues efficiently. It will be the prime responsibility of the researcher to disseminate the correct information to these places of action.

Field personnel consist of a very important group who receive the first-hand experience on what really happens at the ground level. Motivation and awareness among these groups is important. Transmission of their experience, observations, and opinions to the central levels where the decisions are made is important.

Successful disease control depends on an effectively carried out and well-coordinated multidisciplinary action. The clinician, epidemiologist, and the administrator should work together to achieve a mutually shared goal of elimination of leishmaniasis. A multifaceted researcher that looks in to all the related aspects is capable of backing up the operational team with continued search on changing trends.

Several internationally recognized medical schools, well-structured post-graduate training programmes, and paramedical training programmes ensure production of good quality healthcare professionals in Sri Lanka. Quality assurance in training and research is a priority area in these institutions. Health infrastructure covering both curative and preventive aspects is well-organized and fine detailed. Research conducted in many science and technology institutions is supported by many funding and administrative agencies. The literacy rate of the population is high (92%). International transport of infection can be made minimal as Sri Lanka, being an island, is geographically well-separated from other endemic settings. Furthermore, anthroponotic and highly localized nature of the leishmaniasis transmission assures a positive outcome if case detection and treatment are carried out properly.

Tomorrow's researchers on leishmaniasis in Sri Lanka certainly have much in their hands to accomplish. The objectives of this publication are fulfilled if it has left you with insight and interest to do more.

Bibliography

Abeygunasekara PH, et al., *Ceylon Med J* (2007). PMID:17585579/doi:10.4038/cmj. v52i1.1047

Adler S, et al., *Trans R Soc Trop Med Hyg* (1966). PMID:5919627/doi:10.1016/0035-9203 (66)90305-1

Alam MS, et al., *BMC Veterinary Research* (2011). PMCID:PMC3125318/doi:10.1186/ 1746-6148-7-27

Alam MZ, et al., *Infect Genet Evol* (2014). PMID:24480049/doi:10.1016/j.meegid.2014. 01.019

Alam MZ, et al., *Microbes Infect* (2009). PMID:19376262/doi:10.1016/j.micinf.2009. 04.009

Allahverdiyev AM, et al., *Am J Trop Med Hyg* (2004). PMID:15031519/doi:10.4269/ ajtmh.2004.70.294

Allen S, et al., *Leishmaniasis* (1989). doi:10.1007/978-1-4613-1575-9_88

Al-Tawfiq JA, et al., *Int J Infect Dis* (2004). PMID:15234329/doi:10.1016/j. ijid.2003.10.006

Alvar J, et al., *PLoS One* (2012). PMCID:PMC3365071/doi:10.1371/journal.pone.0035671

Amin TT, et al., *Asian Pac J of Trop Med* (2013). PMID:23790342/doi:10.1016/ S1995-7645(13)60116-9

Amit A, et al., *Mol Immunol* (2017). PMID:28064069/doi:10.1016/j.molimm.2016. 12.022

Antonelli LR, et al., *Immuno Lett* (2005). PMID:16083969/doi:10.1016/j.imlet.2005.06.004

Arudpragasam KD, (1982). http://dl.nsf.ac.lk/bitstream/handle/1/5162/NA%20_82. pdf?sequence=1&isAllowed=y

Athukorale DN, et al., *J Trop Med Hyg* (1992). PMID:1460704

Badaro R, et al., *J Infect Dis* (1986). PMID:3782864/doi:10.1093/infdis/154.6.1003

Baldi L, et al., *Parassitologia* (2004). PMID:15305720

Banuls AL, et al., *Adv Parasitol* (2007). PMID:17499100/doi:10.1016/S0065-308X(06) 64001-3

Bates PA, *Int J Parasitol* (2007). PMCID:PMC2675784/doi:10.1016/j.ijpara.2007.04.003

Ben-Ami R, et al., *J Infect* (2002). PMID:12099746/oi:10.1053/jinf.2002.0953

Bern C, et al., *Am J Trop Med Hyg* (2000). PMID:11388512/doi:10.4269/ajtmh.2000. 63.184

Bern C, et al., *PloS Negl Trop Dis* (2008). PMCID:PMC2569207/doi:10.1371/journal. pntd.0000313

Bhandari GP, et al., *Nepal Med Coll J* (2011). PMID:22808821

Bhattacharya SK, et al., *Indian J Med Res* (2006). PMID:16778303

Bhattacharyya T, et al., *PloS Negl Trop Dis* (2013). PMCID:PMC3585016/doi:10.1371/ journal.pntd.0002057

Bhattacharyya T, et al., *PloS Negl Trop Dis* (2014). PMCID:PMC3930516/doi:10.1371/ journal.pntd.0002675

Blackwell JM, et al., *Clin Microbiol Rev* (2009). PMCID:PMC2668228/doi:10.1128/CMR.00048-08

Blum-Domínguez SDC, et al., *Gac Med Mex* (2017). PMID:28128815

Bottrel RLA, et al., *Infect Immun* (2001). PMCID:PMC98281/doi:10.1128/IAI.69.5.3232-3239.2001

Bousoffara T, et al., *J Infect Dis* (2004). PMID:15031796/doi:10.1086/382031

Bridger, J.F.E, 1928. Education, Science and Art. Ceylon Administration Reports. Sri Lanka. Government Printer, Ceylon. C–103

Briercliffe, R., 1930. Education, Science and Art. Ceylon Administration Reports. Sri Lanka. Government Printer, Ceylon. C–32

Brunetti E, *The fauna of British India, including Ceylon and Burma. Diptera Nematocera: Excluding Chironomidae and Culicidae*, (Taylor and Francis, 1912).

Bucheton B, et al., *Am J Hum Genet* (2003). PMCID:PMC1180485/doi:10.1086/379084

Bucheton B, et al., *Microbes Infect* (2002). PMID:12475635/doi:10.1016/s1286-4579(02)00027-8

Cabrera M, et al., *J Exp Med* (1995). PMCID:PMC2192198/doi:10.1084/jem.182.5.1259

Carter HF, et al., *Ann Trop Med Parasitol* (1949). PMID:18121271/doi:10.1080/00034983.1949.11685395

Carvalho LMV, et al., *Rev Inst Med Trop São Paulo* (2017). PMCID:PMC5459540/doi:10.1590/S1678-9946201759033

Castellani A *J Trop Med* (1904).

Castellucci LC, et al., *Mem Inst Oswaldo Cruz* (2014). PMCID:PMC4131779/doi:10.1590/0074-0276140028

Center for leishmaniasis, Faculty of medicine, University of Colombo (2022). https://med.cmb.ac.lk/parasitology/pdru/leishmaniasis/ctrdl/

Cerf BJ, et al., *The J Infect Dis* (1987). PMID:3680989/doi:10.1093/infdis/156.6.1030

Çetin H et al., *Turkiye Parazitol Derg* (2017). PMID:28695834/doi:10.5152/tpd.2017.5296

Chakrabarty R, et al., *J Parasitol* (1996). PMID:8691373

Chakravarty J, et al., *J Glob Infect Dis* (2010). PMCID:PMC2889657/doi:10.4103/0974-777X.62887

Chakravarty J, et al., *PLoS Negl Trop Dis* (2019). PMCID:PMC6453476/doi:10.1371/journal.pntd.0007216

Chamika I, et al., *BMC Infect Dis* (2017). PMCID:PMC5540292/doi:10.1186/s12879-017-2639-7

Chance ML, et al., *Ann Trop Med Parasitol* (1974). PMID:4447389/doi:10.1080/00034983.1974.11686953

Chang KP, Kolli B.K., Collaborators. Overview of Leishmaniasis with Special Emphasis on Kala-azar in South Asia. In: Singh S. (eds) *Neglected Tropical Diseases - South Asia. Neglected Tropical Diseases*, (Springer, Cham, 2017) doi:10.1007/978-3-319-68493-2_1

Chapman RL, *Proc R Soc Med* (1973). PMCID:PMC1645196

Chappuis F, et al., *Nat Rev Microbiol* (2007). PMID:17938629/doi:10.1038/nrmicro1748

Charmoy M, et al., *J Leukoc Biol* (2007). PMID:17449725/doi:10.1189/jlb.0706440

Chowdhury R, et al., *PLoS Negl Trop Dis* (2014). PMCID:PMC4140646/doi:10.1371/journal.pntd.0003020

Clements MF, et al., *Am J Trop Med Hyg* (2010). PMCID:PMC2861389/doi:10.4269/ajtmh.2010.09-0336

Copeland HW, et al., *Am J Trop Med Hyg* (1990). PMID:2221220/doi:10.4269/ajtmh. 1990.43.257

Cupolillo E, et al., *Mol Biochem Parasitol* (1995). PMID:8577322/doi:10.1016/ 0166-6851(95)00108-D

Custodio E, et al., *PloS Negl Trop Dis* (2012). PMCID:PMC3459849/doi:10.1371/ journal.pntd.0001813

Cuypers B, et al., *Infect Genet Evol* (2018). PMCID:PMC6261844/doi:10.1016/j.meegid. 2018.04.021

Darcis G, et al., *BMC Infect Dis* (2017). doi:10.1186/s12879-017-2571-x

Das VNR, et al., *PLoS Negl Trop Dis* (2020). PMCID:PMC7326279/doi:10.1371/ journal.pntd.0008272

Davis JS, et al., *PloS Negl Trop Dis* (2013). PMCID:PMC3772049/doi:10.1371/journal. pntd.0002387

de Almeida MC, *Trends Parasitol* (2002). PMID:11998699/doi:10.1016/s1471-4922(01) 02227-9

de Silva G, et al., *PLoS One* (2017). PMCID:PMC5685575/doi:10.1371/journal. pone.0187024

Dedet JP, Pratlong F, Leishmaniasis In: Cook GC, Zumla AI, (eds) *Manson's Tropical Diseases* (2009).

Deepachandi B et al., *Biomed Res Int* (2020). Article ID:5271657/doi:10.1155/2020/ 5271657

Deepachandi B, *BMC Infect Dis* (2019). PMCID:PMC6631494/doi:10.1186/ s12879-019-4180-3

Deepachandi B, et al., *Int J Anal Chem* (2020). Article ID:6129132/doi:10.1155/2020/ 6129132

Deepachandi B, et al., *Int J Anal Chem* (2020). Article ID:9289651/doi:10.1155/2020/ 9289651

Deepachandi MAB, et al., *The need for continued awareness raising on cutaneous leishmaniasis in Sri Lanka: a case series. Annual Research symposium,* (University of Colombo, 2017).

Desjeux P, Trans R *Soc Trop Med Hyg* (2001). PMID:11490989/doi:10.1016/ s0035-9203(01)90223-8

Desjeux P, *World Health Stat Q* (1992). PMID:1462660

Dey T, et al., *J Eukaryot Microbiol* (2002). PMID:12188216/doi:10.1111/j.1550-7408. 2002.tb00369.x

Dhiman RC, et al., *Infect Dis Poverty* (2016). PMCID:PMC5098277/doi:10.1186/ s40249-016-0200-3

Diniz JLCP, et al., *Braz J Otorhinolaryngol* (2011). PMID:21739015/doi:10.1590/ S1808-86942011000300018

Dissanaike AS, *Soc Protozool, USA* (1981).

Dujardin, JC *Trends Parasitol* (2006). PMID:16300999/doi:10.1016/j.pt.2005.11.004

Ejghal R, et al., *Acta Trop* (2014). PMID:25151047/doi:10.1016/j.actatropica.2014. 08.013

Elamin EM, et al., *Trans R Soc Trop Med Hyg* (2008). PMID:18037149/doi:10.1016/j. trstmh.2007.10.005

El-Hassan AM, et al., *Acta Tropica* (1993). PMID:7903141/doi:10.1016/0001- 706x(93)90051-c

El-Safi SH, *Microbes and Infect* (2002). PMID:12475634/doi:10.1016/S1286-4579(02)
00026-6

El-Tai NO, et al., *Trans R Soc Trop Med Hyg* (2000). PMID:11132393/doi:10.1016/
s0035-9203(00)90093-2

Erber AC, et al., *PLoS Negl Trop Dis* (2020). PMCID:PMC7058360/doi:10.1371/jour-
nal.pntd.0007996

Faber WR, et al., *Clin Exp Dermatol* (2009). PMID:19077092/doi:10.1111/
j.1365-2230.2008.02996.x

Faber WR, et al., *J Am Acad Dermatol* (2003). PMID:12833011/doi:10.1067/mjd.2003.492

Faculty of Medicine, University of Colombo. *National action plan for leishmaniasis
control in Sri Lanka.* (First international colloquium on leishmaniasis, Colombo,
Sri Lanka, 2009).

Flaig MJ, et al., *Br J Dermatol* (2007). PMID:17714564/doi:10.1111/j.1365-2133.
2007.08129.x

Gajapathy K, et al., *Acta Tropica* (2016). PMID:27180216/doi:10.1016/j.actatropica.
2016.05.001

Gajapathy K, et al., *Trop Biomed* (2011). PMID:22041744

Gajapathy K. et al., *Parasit Vectors* (2013). PMCID:PMC3853795/doi:10.1186/1756-
3305-6-302

Galgamuwa LS, et al,. *Parasit Vectors* (2018). PMCID:PMC5785883/doi:10.1186/
s13071-018-2647-5

Galgamuwa LS, et al., *BMC Microbiol* (2019). PMCID:PMC6332851/doi:10.1186/
s12866-018-1384-4

Galgamuwa LS, et al., *Korean J Parasitol* (2017). PMCID:PMC5365259/doi:10.3347/
kjp.2017.55.1.1

Gebre-Michael T, et al., *Med Vet Entomol* (1996). PMID:8834743/doi:10.1111/j.1365-
2915.1996.tb00082.x

Gedda MR, et al., *PLoS Negl Trop Dis* (2020). PMCID:PMC7332242/doi:10.1371/
journal.pntd.0008221

Ghosh SK, et al., *J Indian Med Assoc* (2011). PMID:22666931

González C, et al., *PLoS Negl Trop Dis* (2010). PMCID:PMC2799657/doi:10.1371/
journal.pntd.0000585

Guimarães LH, et al., *PloS Negl Trop Dis* (2016). PMCID:PMC5131895/doi:10.1371/
journal.pntd.0005100

Gunaratna G, et al., *Parasit Vectors* (2018). PMCID:PMC6303884/doi:10.1186/
s13071-018-3238-1

Gunathilaka N, et al., *Biomed Res Int* (2020). PMCID:PMC7453272/doi:10.1155/2020/
5458063

Gunathilaka N, et al., *Parasit Vectors* (2020). PMCID:PMC7236442/doi:10.1186/
s13071-020-04137-8

Gurunath U, et al., *Expert Rev Anti Infect Ther* (2014). PMID:24930676/doi:10.1586/1
4787210.2014.928590

Hadighi R, et al., *PLoS Med* (2006). PMCID:PMC1435779/doi:10.1371/journal.
pmed.0030162

Hanly MG et al., *Cent Afr J Med* (1998). PMID:10101420

Harms G, et al., *Emerg Infect Dis* (2003). PMCID:PMC3023440/doi:10.3201/eid0907.
030023

Hartzell JD, et al., *Am J Trop Med Hyg* (2008). PMID:19052290/doi:10.4269/
ajtmh.2008.79.843

Hasker E, et al., *PLoS Negl Trop Dis* (2014). PMCID:PMC3900391/doi:10.1371/journal.pntd.0002657

Hassan MM, et al., *Parasites Vectors* (2009). PMCID:PMC2706818/doi:10.1186/1756-3305-2-26

Herath CHP, et al., *Ceylon Med J* (2010), PMID:21341622/doi:10.4038/cmj.v55i4.2626

Hewawasam C, et al., *BMC Public Health* (2020). PMCID:PMC7290071/doi:10.1186/s12889-020-09066-w

Hide M, et al., *Acta Trop* (2007). PMID:17544353/doi:10.1016/j.actatropica.2007.04.015

Hirve S, et al., *PLoS Negl Trop Dis* (2017). PMCID:PMC5638223/doi:10.1371/journal.pntd.0005889

Ho TS, et al., *J Biomed Sci* (2013). PMCID:PMC4015130/doi:10.1186/1423-0127-20-75

Hoover DL et al., *J Immunol* (1984). PMID:6363543

Ibrahim ME et al., *Am J Trop Med Hyg* (1999). PMID:10674674/doi:10.4269/ajtmh.1999.61.941

Iddawela D, et al., *BMC Infect Dis* (2018). PMCID:PMC5838877/doi:10.1186/s12879-018-2999-7

Iftikhar N, et al., *Int J Dermatol* (2003). PMID:14521695/doi:10.1046/j.1365-4362.2003.02015.x

Ihalamulla RL et al., *Cey Med J* (2002). PMID:12140880/doi:10.4038/cmj.v47i2.3454

Ihalamulla RL, *Ann of Trop Med Parasitol* (2008). PMID:18318939/doi:10.1179/136485908X252331

Ihalamulla RL, et al., *Ann Trop Med Parasitol* (2005). PMID:16156970/doi:10.1179/136485905X51364

Ihalamulla RL, et al., *Ann Trop Med Parasitol* (2006). PMID:16417718/doi:10.1179/atm.2006.100.1.87

Ihalamulla RL, et al., *Ceylon Med J* (2009). PMID:19670547/doi:10.4038/cmj.v54i2.864

Ihalamulla RL, et al., *Trans R S Trop Med Hyg* (2004). PMID:15109557/doi:10.1016/j.trstmh.2003.10.004

Ilango K, et al., *Ann Trop Med Parasitol* (1994). PMID:7979629/doi:10.1080/00034983.1994.11812884

Ilango K, *J Med Entomol* (2010). PMID:20180302/doi:10.1603/033.047.0101

Imamura H, et al., *eLife* (2016). PMCID:PMC4811772/doi:10.7554/eLife.12613

Ito K, et al., *J Dermatol* (2014). PMID:25228325/doi:10.1111/1346-8138.12609

Jambulingam P, et al., *Acta Trop* (2017). PMID:28327413/doi:10.1016/j.actatropica.2017.03.006

Jamjoom MB, et al., *Parasitology* (2004). PMID:15521628/doi:10.1017/s0031182004005955

Johnson RN, et al., *Trans R Soc Trop Med Hyg* (1993). PMID:8337711/doi:10.1016/0035-9203(93)90461-X

Kahandawaarachchi ICI, et al., *BMC Infect Dis* (2017). PMCID:PMC5540292/doi:10.1186/s12879-017-2639-7

Kalra NL, et al., *J Commun Dis* (1986). PMID:3528275

Kaluarachchi TDJ, et al., *Pathog Glob Health* (2019). PMCID:PMC6758699/doi:10.1080/20477724.2019.1650228

Karakus M, et al., *J Arthropod Borne Dis* (2017). PMCID:PMC5629309

Kariyawasam KKGDUL, et al., *Pathog Glob Health* (2015). PMCID:PMC4768624/doi:10.1179/2047773215Y.0000000032

Kariyawasam UL, et al., *BMC Infect Dis* (2017). doi:10.1186/s12879-017-2883-x

Karunaweera ND, et al., *Sri Lanka Prescriber* (2013).

Karunaweera ND, *Trop Parasitol* (2016). PMCID:PMC4778179/doi:10.4103/2229-5070.175023

Karunaweera, ND et al., *Trans R Soc Trop Med Hyg* (2003). PMID:15259461/doi:10.1016/s0035-9203(03)90061-7

Kaul SM, et al., *J Commun Dis* (1994). PMID:7989678

Killick-Kendrick R, A report presented at the Imperial College at Silwood Park, UK (1996).

Kothalawala HS, et al., *Ceylon Med J* (2016). PMCID:PMC6206497/doi:10.4038/cmj.v61i2.8286

Kuhls K, et al., *Microbes Infect* (2005). PMID:16002315/doi:10.1016/j.micinf.2005.04.009

Kuhls K, et al., *PLoS Negl Trop Dis* (2008). PMCID:PMC2438616/doi:10.1371/journal.pntd.0000261

Kumar NP, et al., *J Med Microbiol* (2015). PMID:25480880/doi:10.1099/jmm.0.076695-0

Kumar R, et al., *Front Immunol* (2012). PMCID:PMC3418610/doi:10.3389/fimmu.2012.00251

Lachaud L, et al., *J Clin Microbiol* (2001). PMCID:PMC87785/doi:10.1128/JCM.39.2.613-617.2001

Lane RP, et al., *J Commun Dis* (1980). PMID:7320487

Lane RP, et al., *Med Vet Entomol* (1990). PMID:2132972/doi:10.1111/j.1365-2915.1990.tb00263.x

Lane RP, et al., *Syst Entomol* (1986). doi:10.1111/j.1365-3113.1986.tb00535.x

Lane RP, *Geographic variation in old world Phlebotomine sandflies*, (Oxford University Press, UK, 1988).

Lang T, et al., *Infect Immun* (2003). PMCID:PMC153224/doi:10.1128/iai.71.5.2674-2683.2003

Lara ML, et al., *Hum Immunol* (1991). PMID:2022495/doi:10.1016/0198-8859(91)90081-j

Laskay T, et al., *Eur J Immunol* (1995). PMID:7664785/doi:10.1002/eji.1830250816

Le Rutte EA, et al., *Epidemics* (2017) PMCID:PMC5340844/doi:10.1016/j.epidem.2017.01.002

Lewis DJ, et al., *Trans R Soc Trop Med Hyg* (1973). PMID:4777431/doi:10.1016/0035-9203(73)90258-7

Lewis DJ, *Syst. Entomol* (1978). doi:10.1111/j.1365-3113.1987.tb00194.x

Lima MHF, et al., *Front Immunol* (2017). PMCID:PMC5517451/doi:10.3389/fimmu.2017.00815

Lira R, et al., *J Infect Dis* (1999). PMID:10395884/doi:10.1086/314896

Loo WJ, et al., *Br J Dermatol* (2005). PMID:16225635/doi:10.1111/j.1365-2133.2005.06921.x

Lukes J, et al., *Proc Natl Acad Sci U S A* (2007). PMCID:PMC1890502/doi:10.1073/pnas.0703678104

Lypaczewski P, et al., *PLoS Negl Trop Dis* (2021). PMCID:PMC7901767/doi:10.1371/journal.pntd.0009079

Lypaczewski P, *Sci Rep* (2018). PMCID:PMC6224596/doi:10.1038/s41598-018-34812-x

Magalhães FB, et al., *PLoS One* (2017). PMCID:PMC5619722/doi:10.1371/journal.pone.0184867

Mahdi M, et al., *Infect Genet Evol* (2005). PMID:15567136/doi:10.1016/j.meegid.2004.05.008

Maia-Elkhoury ANS, et al., *Revista de Saúde Pública* (2007). PMID:18066464/doi:10.1590/s0034-89102007000600007

Manamperi NH, et al., *Am J Trop Med Hyg* (2018). PMCID:PMC5930914/doi:10.4269/ajtmh.17-0748

Manamperi NH, et al., *Parasit Immunol* (2017). PMCID:PMC5354984/doi:10.1111/pim.12413

Marty P, et al., *Ann Trop Med Parasitol* (2007). PMID:17877875/doi:10.1179/136485907X229121

Mary C, et al., *Am J Trop Med Hyg* (1992). PMID:1281966/doi:10.4269/ajtmh.1992.47.764

Massamba NN, et al., *Acta Tropica* (1998). PMID:9879738/doi:10.1016/s0001-706x(98)00071-0

Matlashewski G, et al., *Lancet Glob Health* (2014). PMID:25433617/doi:10.1016/S2214-109X(14)70318-3

Mauricio IL, et al., *Parasitology* (2001). PMID:11315172/doi:10.1017/s0031182001007466

Mauricio IL, et al., *Parasitology* (2004). PMID:15074875/doi:10.1017/s0031182003004578

Maurya R, et al., *J Clin Microbiol* (2010). PMCID:PMC2863905/doi:10.1128/JCM.01733-09

McCall LI, et al., *PLoS Pathog* (2013). PMCID:PMC3536654/doi:10.1371/journal.ppat.1003053

Mebrahtu YB, et al., *Trans R Soc Trop Med Hyg* (1993). PMID:8266420/doi:10.1016/0035-9203(93)90101-U

Mehrotra S, et al., *BMC Med Genet* (2011). PMCID:PMC3260103/doi:10.1186/1471-2350-12-162

Meireles CB, et al., *Acta Trop* (2017). PMID:28526427/doi:10.1016/j.actatropica.2017.05.022

Ministry of Health Sri Lanka Colombo: Epidemiology Unit, (2013) http://www.epid.gov.lk/web/attachments/article/188/Vol%2039%20NO%2002%20 English.pdf

Mishra A, et al., *PLoS One* (2015). PMCID:PMC4420251/doi:10.1371/journal.pone.0124559

Mohamed HS, et al., *Eur J Hum Genet* (2004). PMID:14523377/doi:10.1038/sj.ejhg.5201089

Mohapatra S, *Trop Parasitol* (2014). PMCID:PMC3992802/doi:10.4103/2229-5070.129142

Mollinedo F, et al., *J Biol Chem* (2010). PMCID:PMC2966068/doi:10.1074/jbc.M110.125302

Mondal D, et al., *PLoS Negl Trop Dis* (2009). PMCID:PMC2607537/doi:10.1371/journal.pntd.0000355

Moreno G, et al., Le complexe Leishmania donovani s.l.; Analyse enzymatique et traitement numerique. Individualisation du complexe Leishmania infantum. Corollaires biogeographiques et phyletiques, apropos de 146 souches originaires de l'Ancien et du Nouveau Monde. In: *Leishmania, Taxonomie phylogenese*, (IMEEE, Montpellier, 1986).

Moreno G, Les complexes Leishmania donovani et Leishmania infantum. Implications taxinomiques, biogéographiques et épidémiologiques. A propos de l' analyse enzymatique de 548 souches de l'Ancien et du Nouveau Monde, PhD diss., University of Montpellier (1989).

Moreno I, et al., *Microbes Infect* (2007). PMID:18023393/doi:10.1016/j. micinf.2007.09.009

Mosleh IM, et al., *Trop Med Int Health* (2008). PMID:18363585/doi:10.1111/ j.1365-3156.2008.02063.x

Mouri O, et al., *BMC Infect Dis* (2015). PMCID:PMC4619209/doi:10.1186/s12879-015-1191-6

Muller KH, et al., *Med Microbiol Immunol* (2001). PMID:11770115/doi:10.1007/ s004300100084

Muniaraj M, Trop Parasitol (2014). PMCID:PMC3992795/doi:10.4103/2229-5070. 129143

Murphy ML, et al., *Eur J Immunol* (2001). PMID:11592059/doi:10.1002/1521-4141(2001010)31:10<2848::aid-immu2848>3.0.co;2-t

Murray HW, et al., *J Infect Dis* (2003). PMID:12870129/doi:10.1086/376510

Nadim A, et al., *Trop Geogr Med* (1970). PMID:5497382

Naotunne TD, et al., *Trop Geogr Med* (1990). PMID:2260200

Navin TR, et al., *J Infect Dis* (1992). PMID:1311351/doi:10.1093/infdis/165.3.528

Nawaratna SSK, et al., *Emerg Infect Dis* (2007). PMCID:PMC2878215/doi:10.3201/ eid1307.060773

Nawaratna SSK, et al., *Int J Infect Dis* (2009). PMID:19095480/doi:10.1016/j.ijid.2008. 08.023

Ostyn B, et al., *PLoS Negl Trop Dis* (2011). PMCID:PMC3186756/doi:10.1371/jour-nal.pntd.0001284

Ostyn B, et al., *Trop Med Int Health* (2008). PMID:18564350/doi:10.1111/j.1365-3156. 2008.02110.x

Ozbel Y, et al., *J Vector Ecol* (2011). PMID:21366784/doi:10.1111/j.1948-7134. 2011.00115.x

Pagheh A, et al., *J Parasit Dis* (2014). PMCID:PMC4185041/doi:10.1007/ s12639-013-0316-3

Pandya AP, *Indian J Med Res* (1983). PMID:6674156

Pedral-Sampaio G, et al., *PLoS One* (2016). PMCID:PMC5021300/doi:10.1371/jour-nal.pone.0162793

Perry, A.,1904. Education, Science and Art. Ceylon Administration Reports. Sri Lanka. (Part IV-B). number)

Picado A, et al., *BMJ* (2010). PMCID:PMC3011370/doi:10.1136/bmj.c6760

Poché D, et al., *J Vector Ecol* (2011). PMID:21366762/doi:10.1111/j.1948-7134.2011. 00119.x

Ponce C, et al., *Lancet* (1991). PMID:1670724/doi:10.1016/0140-6736(91)90734-7

Portela ÁSB, et al., *Immunobiology* (2018). PMID:29074301/doi:10.1016/j. imbio.2017.10.043

Pratlong F, et al., *Parasitology* (2001). PMID:11444612/doi:10.1017/S003118200100 7867

Pratlong F, et al., *Trans R Soc Trop Med Hyg* (1995). PMID:7570877/doi:10.1016/ 0035-9203(95)90025-x

Puentes SM, et al., *J Exp Med* (1988). PMCID:PMC2188887/doi:10.1084/jem.167.3.887

Quispe-Tintaya KW, et al., *J Infect Dis* (2005). PMID:16028139/doi:10.1086/432077

Rajapaksa US, et al., *Ceylon Medical Journal* (2005). PMID:16114778

Rajapaksa US, et al., *Trans R Soc Trop Med Hyg* (2007). PMID:17499826/doi:10.1016/j. trstmh.2006.05.013

Ranasinghe S, et al., *Am J Trop Med Hyg* (2013). PMCID:PMC3795106/doi:10.4269/ajtmh.12-0640

Ranasinghe S, et al., *Mem Inst Oswaldo Cruz* (2015). PMCID:PMC4708022/doi:10.1590/0074-02760150286

Ranasinghe S, et al., *Pathog Glob Health* (2012). PMCID:PMC4001626/doi:10.1179/2047773212Y.0000000054

Ranawaka RR, et al., *Ceylon Med J* (2012). PMID:23292056/doi:10.4038/cmj.v57i4.5082

Ranawaka RR, et al., *Int J Dermatol* (2015). PMID:25600472/doi:10.1111/ijd.12685

Ranawaka RR, et al., *J Dermatolog Treat* (2010). PMID:20438389/doi:10.3109/09546630903287445

Ranawaka RR, et al., *J Dermatolog Treat* (2011). PMID:20818996/doi:10.3109/09546631003762654

Ranjan A, et al., *Am J Trop Med Hyg* (2005). PMID:16014837

Rathnayake D, et al., *Int J Dermatol* (2010). PMID:20534090/doi:10.1111/j.1365-4632.2010.04376.x

Reale S, et al., *Transbound Emerg Dis* (2010). PMID:20537100/doi:10.1111/j.1865-1682.2010.01131.x

Refai W et al., *Int J Dermatol* (2019). PMCID:PMC6230306/doi:10.1111/ijd.14240

Refai FW, et al., *Trop Parasitol* (2016). PMCID:PMC5048704/doi:10.4103/2229-5070.190835

Refai W, et al., *Int J Dermatol* (2018). PMCID:PMC6230306/doi:10.1111/ijd.14240

Refai WF, et al., *Am J Trop Med Hyg* (2017). PMCID:PMC5637590/doi:10.4269/ajtmh.16-0879

Reyburn H, et al., *Trans R Soc Trop Med Hyg* (2003). PMID:14584372/doi:10.1016/s0035-9203(03)90111-8

Ribas-Silva RC, et al., *Genet Mol Res* (2015). PMID:26600554/doi:10.4238/2015.November.18.58

Rodgers MR, et al., *Exp Parasitol* (1990). PMID:2170165/doi:10.1016/0014-4894(90)90031-7

Rodrigues V, et al., *Parasit Vectors* (2016). PMCID:PMC4774109/doi:10.1186/s13071-016-1412-x

Rodriguez B, et al., *Parasite Immunol* (2007). PMID:17518946/doi:10.1111/j.1365-3024.2007.00944.x

Rosypal AC, et al., *J Parasitol* (2010). PMID:19803542/doi:10.1645/GE-2288

Roychoudhury J, et al., *Indian J Biochem Biophys* (2008).

Sakthianandeswaren A, et al., *Trends Parasitol* (2009). PMID:19617002/doi:10.1016/j.pt.2009.05.004

Salotra P, et al., *J Clin Microbiol* (2001). PMCID:PMC87840/doi:10.1128/JCM.39.3.849-854.2001

Samaranayake N, et al., *BMC Infect Dis* (2016). PMCID:PMC4908677/doi:10.1186/s12879-016-1626-8

Samaranayake TN, et al., *Ann Trop Med Parasitol* (2008). PMID:18577329/doi:10.1179/136485908X300779

Samaranayake TN, et al., *Trop Med Int Health* (2010). PMID:20214763/doi:10.1111/j.1365-3156.2010.02491.x

Samarasinghe SR, et al., *BMC Genomics* (2018). PMCID:PMC6262978/doi:10.1186/s12864-018-5271-z

Sandanayaka R, et al., *Trop Med Int Health* (2014). PMID:24438012/doi:10.1111/tmi.12232

Sanyal RK, et al., *J Commun Dis* (1979).

Saporito L, et al., *Int J Infect Dis* (2013). PMID:23380419/doi:10.1016/j.ijid.2012.12.024

Sarkari B, et al., *Interdiscip Perspect Infect Dis* (2014). PMCID:PMC4142716/doi:10.1155/2014/505134

Satoskar AR, et al., *J Immunol* (1999). PMID:10553052

Scharton TM, et al., *J Exp Med* (1993). PMCID:PMC2191131/doi:10.1084/jem.178.2.567

Schenkel K, et al., *Trop Med Int Health* (2006). PMID:17176343/doi:10.1111/j.1365-3156.2006.01735.x

Schnur LF, et al., Adult visceral leishmaniasis caused by *Leishmania donovani sensu stricto* acquired locally in Israel. 2nd World Congress on Leishmaniasis, (Hersonissos, Crete, 2001).

Schnur LF, et al., *Ann Trop Med Parasitol* (1977). PMID:921364/doi:10.1080/00034983.1977.11687191

Semage SN, et al., *Int J Infect Dis* (2014). PMID:24858902/doi:10.1016/j.ijid.2014.03.1382

Senanayake SASC, et al., *Southeast Asian J Trop Med Public Health* (2015). PMCID:PMC6206496

Seneviratne JKK, et al., *Kandy Med J* (1995).

Sethuraman G, et al., *N Engl J Med* (2008). PMID:18199877/doi:10.1056/NEJMc072391

Sharma NL, et al., *Am J Trop Med Hyg* (2005). PMID:15964970

Sharma U, et al., *Indian J Exp Biol* (2009). PMID:19634705

Shaw J, *Mem Inst Oswaldo Cruz* (2007). PMID:17899628/doi:10.1590/S0074-02762007000500001

Shirani-Bidabadi L, et al., *Acta Trop* (2017). PMID:28870534/doi:10.1016/j.actatropica.2017.08.035

Silva LA, et al., *Rev Inst Med Trop Sao Paulo* (2013). PMID:23563762/doi:10.1590/S0036-46652013000200006

Silveira FT, et al., *Mem Inst Oswaldo Cruz* (2004). PMID:15273794/doi:10.1590/S0074-02762004000300001

Singh OP, et al., *Clin Infect Dis* (2014). PMCID:PMC4001287/doi:10.1093/cid/ciu102

Singh OP, et al., *J Parasitol Res* (2015). PMCID:PMC4710934/doi:10.1155/2015/239469

Singla N, et al., *FEMS Microbiol Lett* (1992). PMID:1426984/doi:10.1111/j.1574-6968.1992.tb05322.x

Siriwardana HVYD, et al., *Ann Trop Med Parasitol* (2010). PMID:20507695/doi:10.1179/136485910X12647085215615

Siriwardana HVYD, et al., *Biomed Res Int* (2021). Article ID:3537968/doi:10.1155/2021/3537968

Siriwardana HVYD, et al., *Ceylon Med J* (2003). PMID:12795012/doi:10.4038/cmj.v48i1.3386

Siriwardana HVYD, et al., *Emerg Infect Dis* (2007). PMCID:PMC2725894/doi:10.3201/eid1303.060242

Siriwardana HVYD, et al., *Pathog Glob Health* (2015). PMCID:PMC4530555/doi:10.1179/2047773215Y.0000000024

Siriwardana HVYD, et al., *Pathog Glob Health* (2017). PMCID:PMC5694859/doi:10.1080/20477724.2017.1361564

Siriwardana HVYD, et al., *SLJID* (2012). doi:10.4038/sljid.v2i2.4420

Siriwardana HVYD, Studies on the clinical epidemiology of cutaneous leishmaniasis in Sri Lanka, and the molecular identification of the parasite, PhD diss., University of Colombo (2008).

Siriwardana Y, et al., *Biomed Res Int* (2019). PMCID:PMC6487155/doi:10.1155/2019/4093603

Siriwardana Y, et al., *J Trop Med* (2019). PMCID:PMC6556790/doi:10.1155/2019/4538597

Siriwardana Y, et al., *J Trop Med* (2019). PMCID:PMC6683790/doi:10.1155/2019/6475939

Siriwardana YD, et al., *Biomed Res Int* (2018). PMCID:PMC5822831/doi:10.1155/2018/9320367

Srinivasan R, et al., *Acta Trop* (2014). PMID:24832008/doi:10.1016/j.actatropica.2014.04.023

Srivastava P, et al., *Trop Med Int Health* (2013). PMID:23464581/doi:10.1111/tmi.12085

Stauch A, et al., *PLoS Negl Trop Dis* (2011). PMCID:PMC3226461/doi:10.1371/journal.pntd.0001405

Stockdale L, et al., *PLoS Negl Trop Dis* (2013). PMCID:PMC3688540/doi:10.1371/journal.pntd.0002278

Sudarshan M et al., *Diagn Microbiol Infect Dis* (2014). PMCID:PMC4157122/doi:10.1016/j.diagmicrobio.2014.01.031

Sukra K, et al., *Parasitol Res* (2013). PMID:23052769/doi:10.1007/s00436-012-3137-x

Sundar S, et al., *Ann Trop Med Parasitol* (2002). PMID:11989529/doi:10.1179/000349802125000466

Sundar S, et al., *BMJ* (1994). PMCID:PMC2539260/doi:10.1136/bmj.308.6924.307

Sundar S, et al., *Expert Rev Anti Infect Ther* (2018). PMCID:PMC6345646/doi:10.1080/14787210.2018.1532790

Sundar S, et al., *J Clin Microbiol* (2006). PMCID:PMC1351954/doi:10.1128/JCM.44.1.251-253.2006

Sundar S, et al., *Mol Diagn Ther* (2018). PMCID:PMC6301112/doi:10.1007/s40291-018-0343-y

Surendran SN, et al., *Bull Entomol Res* (2005). PMID:16048685/doi:10.1079/ber2005368

Surendran SN, et al., *J Vector Borne Dis* (2005). PMID:16457386

Surendran SN, et al., *J Vector Borne Dis* (2007). PMID:17378219

Svobodová M, et al., *Int J Parasitol* (2009). PMID:18761342/doi:10.1016/j.ijpara.2008.06.016

Swaminath CS, et al., *Indian J Med Res* (2006). PMID:16789343

Szargiki R, et al., *Braz J Infect Dis* (2009). PMID:19578630/doi:10.1590/S1413-86702009000100011

Takagi H, et al., *Am J Trop Med Hyg* (2009). PMID:19815869 doi:10.4269/ajtmh.2009.09-0145

Thakur L, et al., *PLoS Negl Trop Dis* (2018). PMCID:PMC6159859/doi:10.1371/journal.pntd.0006659

Tharmatha T, et al., *Bull Entomol Res* (2017). PMID:27719684/doi:10.1017/S0007485316000626

Tomasini C, et al., *J Cutan Pathol* (2017). PMID:28294400/doi:10.1111/cup.12927

Toz SO, et al., *Trop Med Int Health* (2009). PMID:19737374/doi:10.1111/
j.1365-3156.2009.02384.x

Ulett GC, et al., *Infect Immun* (2000). PMCID:PMC97383 doi:10.1128/iai.68.4.2034-
2042.2000

Uranw S, et al., *BMC Infect Dis* (2013). PMCID:PMC3552873/doi:10.1186/
1471-2334-13-21

Vallur AC, et al., *J Clin Microbiol* (2016). PMCID:PMC4809943 doi:10.1128/
JCM.02620-15

WHO expert committee on the control of the leishmaniases and World Health
Organization, (2010). http://whqlibdoc.who.int/trs/WHO_TRS_949_eng.pdf

Wijerathna T, et al., *Biomed Res Int* (2018). PMCID:PMC6201334/doi:10.1155/
2018/3025185

WijerathnaT,etal.,*ParasitVectors*(2020a).PMCID:PMC7275303/doi:10.1186/s13071-020-
04154-7

Wijerathna T, et al., *Parasit Vectors* (2020b). PMCID:PMC7487486/doi:10.1186/
s13071-020-04305-w

Wijerathna T, et al., *Parasit Vectors* (2020c). PMCID:PMC7216469/doi:10.1186/
s13071-020-04122-1

Wijesinghe H, et al., *Biomed Res Int* (2020). PMCID:PMC7222607/doi:10.1155/2020/
4926819

Wijesundera MS, *Ceylon Med J* (2001). PMID:12164035/doi:10.4038/cmj.v46i4.6467

World Health Organization, (2005). https://apps.who.int/iris/handle/10665/205825

World Health Organization, (2014) https://apps.who.int/iris/bitstream/handle/10665/205826/
B4870.pdf?sequence=1&isAllowed=y

World Health Organization, (2014). http://www.searo.who.int/mediacentre/releases/2014/
pr1581/en/

Yatawara L, et al., *Trop Med Health* (2008). doi:10.2149/tmh.2008-21

Yogeswari S, et al., *J Med Entomol* (2016). PMID:26768941/doi:10.1093/jme/tjv249

Zemanova E, et al., *Am J Trop Med Hyg* (2004). PMID:15211001/doi:10.4269/
ajtmh.2004.70.613

Zeyrek FY, et al., *Clin Vaccine Immunol* (2007). PMCID:PMC2168175/doi:10.1128/
CVI.00133-07

Zhang WW, et al., *J Biol Chem* (2003). PMID:12829719/doi:10.1074/jbc.M305030200

Zhang WW, et al., *PLoS Pathog* (2014). PMCID:PMC4081786 doi:10.1371/journal.
ppat.1004244

Index

Printed in the United States
by Baker & Taylor Publisher Services